Hospice and Palliative Care Acupuncture

of related interest

Acupuncture Strategies for Complex Patients
From Consultation to Treatment
Skya Abbate, DOM
ISBN 978 1 84819 380 2
eISBN 978 0 85701 336 1

Treating Emotional Trauma with Chinese Medicine
Integrated Diagnostic and Treatment Strategies
CT Holman, MS, LAc
ISBN 978 1 84819 318 5
eISBN 978 0 85701 271 5

Treating Body and Soul
A Clinicians' Guide to Supporting the Physical, Mental
and Spiritual Needs of Their Patients
Edited by Peter Wells
ISBN 978 1 78592 148 3
eISBN 978 1 78450 417 5

Psycho-Emotional Pain and the Eight Extraordinary Vessels
Yvonne R. Farrell, DAOM, LAc
ISBN 978 1 84819 292 8
eISBN 978 0 85701 239 5

Hospice *and* Palliative Care
ACUPUNCTURE

TORII BLACK

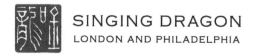

SINGING DRAGON
LONDON AND PHILADELPHIA

The extract from *The Secret of Chinese Pulse Diagnosis* (Flaws 1995) is reprinted with permission from Blue Poppy Press.

Table 9.1: The Functional Assessment Staging Test (FAST) is reproduced with permission from Barry Reisberg, MD.

The treatment protocol on pages 166–9 is reprinted with permission from *Medical Acupuncture* journal (Sudhakaran 2017), published by Mary Ann Liebert, Inc., New Rochelle, NY 10801.

First published in 2020
by Singing Dragon
an imprint of Jessica Kingsley Publishers
73 Collier Street
London N1 9BE, UK
and
400 Market Street, Suite 400
Philadelphia, PA 19106, USA

www.singingdragon.com

Copyright © Torii Black 2020

Front cover image source: Shutterstock°.

Library of Congress Cataloging in Publication Data
A CIP catalog record for this book is available from the Library of Congress

British Library Cataloguing in Publication Data
A CIP catalogue record for this book is available from the British Library

ISBN 978 1 84819 421 2
eISBN 978 0 85701 373 6

Printed and bound by CPI Group (UK) Ltd, Croydon, CR0 4YY

3

Contents

1. Introduction   9

2. Hospice and Palliative Care History and Philosophy . . .   13
   What is a hospice and where did it come from?   13
   Spiritual considerations.   14
   Death moves from family care to hospital   15
   The nurse who became a Dame   16
   An American counterpart   17
   An abbreviated history of hospice in the United States   18

3. Chinese Culture Influences on Modern Death and Dying
   Issues   25
   The search for longevity   25
   The family   26
   After the patient dies   27
   Hospice and palliative care in China   28

4. East Meets West—The Face of Modern Palliative Care . .   31
   What about acupuncture?   32
   Research and cost effectiveness   34
   Growth potential for hospice and palliative care.   35
   Who pays for hospice?   36
   Who regulates hospices?   37
   How does hospice work?   37

The Palliative Performance Scale 38

Why hospice, why now? 39

The interdisciplinary team 42

Other therapies offered by modern hospices. 45

5. Integrating Acupuncture into Current Hospice and
   Palliative Care Models 49

   What does acupuncture do, or how does it work?. 51

   Does it hurt? 53

   How many needles do you use? 54

   How many treatments does it require to be effective?. 54

   Does insurance cover it, or how do you get paid for treatments?
   54

   What can you use acupuncture for in palliative care? 55

   What can you use acupuncture for in hospice and palliative
   care? 57

6. Assessment, Diagnosis, and Treatment of the Patients at
   the End of Life 63

   An emotional perspective on grief 63

   Diagnosis by looking 65

   Diagnosis by hearing and smelling 70

   Diagnosis by asking. 71

   Diagnosis by feeling 74

   Pulse diagnosis 75

   Another view from the Golden Mirror 78

7. Five Elements 81

   Water 82

   Wood 83

   Metal 83

   Earth 83

   Fire 84

   Principles of treatment 84

   Treatment techniques. 86

   Hospice Acupuncture Protocol 86

8. Channel Points for Consideration 93

Wood 93

Fire 95

Earth 100

Metal 103

Water 107

Other points 112

9. The Major Hospice Diagnoses 115

What are the major hospice diagnoses? 115

Cancer 116

Dementia 128

Heart disease 134

HIV/AIDS 140

Liver disease 150

Neurological disease 161

Pulmonary disease 172

Renal failure 175

Stroke or coma 180

Terminal illness: general (non-specific) 188

The last treatment 194

Conclusion 194

10. Final Thoughts 199

Appendix: NAHPCA Treatment Protocol 201

Glossary for Point Nomenclature 205

References 209

Index 217

Chapter 1

Introduction

L et's start with the facts. Everyone dies. Even though we don't like to talk about it, every year an estimated 55.3 million people in the world die, and 40 million need palliative care (World Health Organization (WHO) 2018a). When asked, the majority of people will tell you that they would prefer to die at home, surrounded by their loved ones. Unfortunately, the truth in some countries is that more than 75 percent of deaths occur in hospitals, assisted living facilities, skilled nursing homes, or other places. Conversely, of the millions of patients who are treated by hospices annually, the majority die at home. In 2011, a study cited by the WHO reported that of 234 countries, territories, and areas reviewed, palliative care services were well integrated in as few as 20 countries, while 42 percent (98) had no palliative care services at all and a further 32 percent (75) had only isolated palliative care services (Lynch, Connor, and Clark 2013).

Unfortunately, even in countries where hospice services are available to all, the majority of terminally ill patients do not understand the services, or don't know about hospices.

Hospice is a calling, and not everyone is suited to it, but now is the time to learn geriatric, palliative care, and hospice acupuncture. The current geriatric population is on the edge of a monumental wave that will affect the face of healthcare worldwide. The baby boomers are the majority of the 617 million people aged 65 and over today, and this group will increase to 1.6 billion by 2050 (National Institute of Health 2016). This group has been one of the largest, most influential groups in the history of the world, and they will be needing and expecting hospice services.

The historical baby boom did not occur worldwide, but most experts agree this post-World War II phenomenon occurred between 1946 and 1964 and lasted for periods of 4–18 years in the US, UK, Canada, Finland, Germany, Sweden, Denmark, the Netherlands, Ireland, Hungary, Iceland, New Zealand, Australia, Japan, Italy, and France. Several factors added to this boom. There was a new optimism based on rebuilding after the end of World War II and the Great Depression. Massive battalions of soldiers were returning home from the war. Contraceptive methods were relatively poor, birth control devices and medications were limited, new, or only available to married women. Abortion was illegal in most countries. A final influence was the (pre-women's movement) cultural belief that women who had been recruited to work for the war effort should return home to fulfill their "natural" roles as wives and mothers, and they should not work outside the home.

This baby boomer generation makes up 15 percent of all the people in the world. By 2030, they will be 20 percent of the population, all between the ages of 65 and 83. An estimated 75 percent of the baby boomers (462.75 million people) suffer from chronic conditions (United States Census Bureau 2009), which means there is and will continue to be a corresponding exponential need for palliative care and for hospice-trained professionals.

Hospice incorporates a team approach to patient care based on treating the whole person. The top nine out of ten causes of death in the world have the potential to have prolonged treatments associated with them (the tenth cause is road accidents) (Mitchell 2017). There is an effective acupuncture protocol that can help people gain physical comfort and resolve deep emotional issues at the end of life. Acupuncture is also helpful for family or loved ones who are suffering with loss and grief.

Despite being safe and cost effective, acupuncture and Asian Medicine treatments are underutilized in hospice and palliative care.[1] There are some admitting providers (doctors who review patients' conditions and approve them for hospice care) who refuse

---

1   Asian Medicine will be used in this book to refer to Oriental Medicine and Traditional Chinese Medicine, unless referenced from another source as a direct quotation.

to refer patients to complementary practitioners. Other obstacles for the inclusion of Asian Medicine as part of palliative care include lack of reimbursement by national health insurance, and, in some areas, a lack of proper credentialing, or no available acupuncture professionals.

Educating yourself about the philosophy, history, structure, and financial aspects of hospices will give you confidence in dealing with hospice organizations in your country or area. You will be able to communicate with hospice professionals and build a referral base to expand your practice or become a "bridge builder" and join an interdisciplinary team.

This book introduces you to cultural, physical, spiritual, and emotional issues related to death and dying. It provides you with assessment and treatment options for patients that will allow them to release these issues and die a peaceful death. By becoming a hospice-certified professional, you are showing your dedication to the advancement of the acupuncture profession as a practitioner integrating Eastern and Western medicine to best serve our patients.

Chapter 2

Hospice and Palliative Care History and Philosophy

For you to be an effective and successful hospice and palliative care practitioner, it is important to understand the history and philosophy of hospices.

What is a hospice and where did it come from?

The modern concept of hospitality—to receive a stranger or guest with liberality and goodwill—has its roots in the 11th century. Hospice is derived from the Latin word *hospitium*—a place for travelers and pilgrims, and just as often for the sick and dying. The structures were usually inns kept by a religious order (Harrison 2008). The word hospice, however, was not meant to define a physical place (like an inn); instead it was meant to represent the spirit of hospitality.

Hospice is a philosophy of care which, akin to modern nursing theory, embraces a holistic view of the patient. It encompasses the whole person, including physical, emotional, and spiritual concerns. Hospice programs are designed to provide care custom-fitted to a patient's living environment, whether that is a private home, an assisted living situation, a skilled nursing care facility, a hospital, or a combination of those places.

The hospice concept of care provides compassion, concern, and support for the dying. Traditionally, an end-of-life prognosis is limited to the projected last six months of life, but the focus is on quality, not quantity, of days. While organized under a variety of models, most hospices make care available to patients and their families 24 hours a day, 7 days a week.

The hospice philosophy:

- is an affirmation of life, dedicated to upholding dignity and the highest quality of life possible in end-of-life situations. It aims at keeping the patient alert and pain free, and allowing them to be surrounded by loved ones

- supports the inevitable conclusion of the journey of life: the understanding that everyone dies. It accepts death as the final stage of life, a stage in which people can continue to grow and teach others as they examine and come to terms with their own beliefs on dying

- encourages patients and families to participate in the plan of care. They are taught options and are educated in signs and symptoms of disease progression. The patient's personal preferences are sought to promote self-determination and appropriate care

- provides an interdisciplinary team of palliative care experts. The team is a supportive group that embraces palliation (managing symptoms and reducing the severity of the disease process, rather than attempting to cure it) as an appropriate model of care.

Adapted from American Cancer Society 2009
and Harrison 2008

Spiritual considerations

Hospice philosophy includes acknowledging and addressing a person's spiritual needs. Some hospices have chaplains on their teams. Most are specially trained in ethnic and religious differences. Spirituality is more than where a patient worships or what their religious affiliation is. Even patients who are not affiliated with a specific religion or denomination may wish to get in touch with their spirituality.

Dying people often search for a meaning and purpose to their existence. This is expressed by a desire to review their lives. Patients may reunite with family members, return to religious services, or participate in other rituals tied to their previous concept of God, or what they perceive as the greater order of life. These acts often reduce fears or bring comfort in the face of the unknown. Conversely, if family members or significant others disagree with the patient's beliefs, it can cause additional stress.

Mother Teresa expressed an understanding of the spiritual partnership that happens when people come together to help a dying person. She is best known for her work among the dying destitute in Calcutta, India. She stated, "Food, shelter, and care are what the dying need, but even greater is their need for being wanted. What you can do, I cannot do, and what I can do, you cannot do. Together we can do something beautiful for God" (cited in Hospice and Palliative Care of Virginia 2009). If you do not believe in God, you could easily substitute the words humankind, love, or greater good to arrive at the same sentiment.

In order to understand the current state of end-of-life care in nations with advanced healthcare, one must look at the history and development of hospice and palliative care.

Death moves from family care to hospital

In our great-grandparents' time, it was commonplace for households to consist of three or more generations. Births and deaths happened in the family home and were viewed as natural events. Rituals around death and dying were often acculturated but not directly taught or discussed.

As modern medicine developed, birth and death were transplanted to hospitals. Doctors became authority figures, and family members became guests with little say in or control of what happened to their loved ones (Hospice and Palliative Care of Virginia 2009). Often the physician's determination—to try to save a patient at all costs and measures—was out of focus with the reality of the patient's prognosis.

A patient who could not be saved was perceived as a failure of modern medicine, instead of an inevitable part of a natural cycle. Death and dying were given less attention in the medical world, which sharpened its focus on improving quality of life, and funded major research projects aimed at curing diseases and extending longevity. Many people with life-limiting diseases were debilitated due to the effects of chronic and acute pain. These patients were prescribed standard pain medication doses that were far below the level needed for comfort. Physicians feared side effects and overdoses because they lacked knowledge regarding drug tolerance and pain management. It was a British nurse, Cicely Saunders, who would start the movement back toward equilibrium, balancing patients' needs with updated medical practices.

The nurse who became a Dame

Cicely Mary Saunders started her journey to fame as a nursing student in England in 1940. In 1944, she returned to St. Anne's College, Oxford, after suffering from a back injury, and completed her BA in 1945. In 1947, she took the exam to qualify as a social worker and became a lady almoner (a hospital social worker) that year at St. Thomas's Hospital in London.

Ten years later, in 1957, at St. Thomas's College, Cicely qualified to become a physician. Dr. Saunders suffered three personal losses in 1960: her father, a good friend, and the man she was in love with. These deaths sent her into a period of what she termed as "pathological grieving."

She spent many of the years between 1957 and 1963 conducting extensive research in pain management. Dr. Saunders focused on the importance of palliative care in modern medicine. In 1963, she delivered her ideas to the United States in a lecture on pain management at Yale University. Her groundbreaking work did not go unnoticed by England's Ministry of Health. In 1965, she was made an Officer of the British Empire.

Two years later, in 1967, Saunders became the medical director of the world's first hospice house built specifically for dying patients, St. Christopher's Hospice in South London. This began a trend of associating the word and philosophy of hospice with a physical building.

St. Christopher's emphasized a combination of exceptional symptom and pain relief backed by clinical research and teaching, offered in a holistic environment. Treatments and visits took into account the patient's spiritual, psychological, and physical condition as well as the social needs of the patient, family, and friends. She saw the patient's process of acceptance as a form of completion. She taught, "We do not have to cure to heal." The early principles of the first modern hospice still stand today.

Dr. Saunders became Dame Cicely in 1979 when she was elevated by knighthood to Dame of the British Empire. In 1985, Dame Saunders took the position of chairwoman at St. Christopher's Hospice, and became president in 2000. She died of cancer five years later, at the age of 87 (Pajka 2017). True to her nature and her beliefs, she died in the hospice that she founded. She will forever be remembered as the founder of the modern hospice movement.

An American counterpart

Florence Wald was an American nurse who became known as "the mother of the American hospice movement." In 1959, she became the Dean of Yale School of Nursing. Four years later, she heard Dr. Saunders' lecture on the hospice practice and philosophy. That lecture drove her to refocus and update the curriculum of the Nursing School. She changed the scope of her teaching to include the patient and their family as active participants in care.

In 1971, inspired by Saunders' work, Wald conducted a two-year study on terminally ill patients. Her central theme was home versus facility care, and how the patients and their families felt about the process. In 1974, she founded the first modern United States hospice program in Branford, Connecticut, but resigned shortly after it was opened.

She remained a champion for the hospice cause. For her pioneering work, she was awarded an honorary doctorate from Yale in 1996. An activist even into her 80s, she served on the board of directors and conducted a research project for the National Prison

Hospice Association. Florence Wald died in 2008 in her home at the age of 91. The roots of her original work spread into a system of care that has helped millions to die with dignity (Pajka 2017).

An abbreviated history of hospice in the United States

As previously stated, palliative care services are not readily available to a large part of the world's population. The WHO report (Connor and Bermedo 2014) lists only the following countries as those where hospice-palliative services are at a stage of advanced integration into mainstream service provision: Australia, Austria, Belgium, Canada, France, Germany, Hong Kong, Iceland, Ireland, Italy, Japan, Norway, Poland, Romania, Singapore, Sweden, Switzerland, Uganda, United Kingdom (UK), and United States (US).

Let's take a look at some of the historical steps and milestones recorded by the National Hospice and Palliative Care Organization. This is a demonstration of 40 years of progress and the political involvement required to get one country to this level of hospice care. The following excerpts from the history of hospice are from two websites, with some duplicate data: National Hospice and Palliative Care Organization 2019 and Hospice Association of America 2009.

1969: Publishing house Macmillan takes a chance and publishes a book by a little-known author, Elisabeth Kübler-Ross. The book, entitled *On Death and Dying*, is based on more than 500 interviews with dying patients.

1972: The first hearing on death and dying with dignity is conducted by the US Senate Special Committee. In her testimony, Elisabeth Kübler-Ross states:

> We live in a very particular death-denying society. We isolate both the dying and the old, and it serves a purpose. They are reminders of our own mortality. We should not institutionalize people. We can give families more help with home care and visiting nurses, giving the families and the patients the spiritual, emotional, and financial

help in order to facilitate the final care at home. (National Hospice and Palliative Care Organization 2019)

1974: The first hospice legislation is introduced (but not enacted) to provide federal funds for hospice programs. The National Cancer Institute funds home care for the Connecticut Hospice.

1977 and 1978: The National Cancer Institute provides funding for additional hospices.

1978: A report is published from the US Department of Health, Education, and Welfare. It considers hospice care to be a viable concept for terminally ill people and their families. The report further finds hospices provide humane care at a reduced cost when compared with nursing home care.

1979: The Administration on Aging funds several hospice demonstration projects to determine what defines hospice and hospice care. The study measures cost effectiveness and helps to determine what a hospice should provide.

1980: Joint Commission on Accreditation of Hospitals (JCAH) gets a grant to investigate the status of hospice and to develop standards for hospice accreditation.

1984: Hospice costs are recognized as significantly less than conventional care costs for lengths of stay lasting less than two months. The National Hospice Study labels hospice care as a viable and medically sound alternative to conventional care. JCAH initiates hospice accreditation.

1986: Congress makes the Medicare Hospice Benefit permanent. Hospices are given a 10 percent increase in reimbursement rates, and care is made available to terminally ill patients in nursing homes. State Medicaid programs are given the option of including hospice services.

1991: The National Defense Authorization Act enables hospice care in military hospitals and under TRICARE. The Commission on the Future Structure of Veterans Health Care and the Hospice Association of America (HAA) recommend including hospice care in the veterans' benefit package.

1993: Hospice is included as a nationally guaranteed benefit under President Clinton's healthcare reform proposal. More than 1288 hospices participate in the Medicare program, making it an accepted part of the healthcare continuum.

1994: A provision in the Social Security Act Amendments requires patients being discharged from a hospital to have a planner "evaluate a patient's likely need for appropriate post-hospital services, including hospice services and the availability of those services."

1995: Hospice Interpretive Guidelines for participating programs are expanded for clarification. The Civilian Health and Medical Program of the Uniformed Services (CHAMPUS) hospice benefit is implemented. It mirrors the Medicare hospice benefit in Conditions of Participation and reimbursement.

1996: The Volunteer Hospice Network (VHN), a national forum for volunteer hospices, is created by the HAA. Hospices meet to share information and resources. Through information sharing, they develop ways to cooperate with Medicare-certified hospices and to expand their own services.

The same year the Ninth US Circuit Court of Appeals in San Francisco and the Second US Circuit Court of Appeals overturn laws against physician-assisted suicide. Both rulings are appealed to the US Supreme Court.

1997: The US Supreme Court rules against physician-assisted suicide. It rules that mentally competent terminally ill people do not have that right under the constitution. Congress further forbids the use of taxpayer dollars for financing physician-assisted suicide. In a state decision, Oregon voters pass the "Death with Dignity Act," allowing physician-assisted suicide.

2000: Congress approves an increase of the base payment in the Medicare Hospice Benefit.

2003: Congress passes the Medicare Prescription Drug, Improvement, and Modernization Act of 2003 (HR 1 and S 1). Hospices gain three important benefits: 1) they can authorize payment for hospice palliative care consultations; 2) nurse practitioners can now follow their patients onto the hospice benefit; and 3) hospices can contract for highly specialized nursing services, and contract with other hospices.

2005: Hospice Conditions of Participation are printed in the Federal register with newly proposed updates.

2007: Change Request 5567 is issued by the Centers for Medicare and Medicaid Services (CMS). It requires hospices to bill and report all visits and charges of physicians and nurse practitioners acting as attending physicians, nurses, social workers, and home aides. CMS grants a six-month extension ordering it into effect in January 2008. Templates are developed to help hospices create standard charges per visit.

2008: The Medicare Hospice Benefit final Conditions of Participation are released. This is the first major rewrite since 1983, when the benefit began.

2009: *The NHPCO Standards of Practice for Pediatric Palliative Care and Hospice,* along with the companion publication *Facts and Figures on Pediatric Palliative and Hospice Care in America,* are released. *Quality Guidelines for Hospice and End-of-Life Care in Correctional Settings* is published by NHPCO.

2010: The Patient Protection and Affordable Care Act is passed by the Congress. A provision requires state Medicaid programs to allow children with a life-limiting illness to receive both hospice care and curative treatment.

2013: ehospice is launched as a globally run online news and information resource committed to offering the latest news, commentary, and analysis from the world of hospice and palliative care. ehospiceUSA is powered by NHPCO.

2016: CMS launches hospice payment reform—the first change to the Medicare hospice payment system since the benefit was established.

2018: The Medicare Patient Access to Hospice Act was signed by the President in February.

- Legislation was passed to address the Opioid crisis, including a safe disposal provision for qualified hospice staff.

Hospice has evolved from volunteer and grassroots organizations in the 1970s to the multimillion-dollar healthcare companies of today. Modern hospices are regulated to provide quality practices and are funded to support professional staff. Whether profit or non-profit, independent or part of a health system or hospital, there were 4382 Medicare-certified hospices in the US in 2016, serving more than 1.43 million people that year (National Hospice and Palliative Care Organization 2017).

There is another important piece of this healthcare puzzle—the rising number of home deaths. In the US, the category "hospice" wasn't included on death certificates until a revised death certificate was issued in 2003. The number of patients who died at home under hospice care was not recorded, or they were simply recorded as a home death. Statistics for hospice deaths are still skewed, as the numbers of states using the new certificate grew from four states in 2003 to 46 states and the District of Columbia in 2014.

According to the Centers for Disease Control and Prevention report in 2016, the number of deaths that occurred in a hospital decreased 25.7 percent from approximately half (50.2%) in 2000 to 37.3 percent in 2014. Deaths in a nursing home or long-term care facility decreased by 10.1 percent during the years 2005–14. The percentage of deaths that occurred at the decedent's home increased by 29.5 percent in the 14-year period from 2000 to 2014. Deaths that occurred in hospice and all other places increased from 3.5 percent in 2000 to 12 percent in 2014. It is important to note that these hospice death numbers did not count patients who were receiving hospice care while in hospitals, nursing or long-term care, or assisted living facilities, so again, the influence of hospice care is under-reported.

The baby boomers have lived well and expect to die well. For many people, dying well means a home death with loved ones present. Many boomers have embraced acupuncture, and want it to be part of their healthcare, or for it to be made available for their parents or children who are dying. In 2016, there were 1.43 million hospice patients in America. It is one of the fastest-growing healthcare specialties in the world. Even if you don't plan on making it your specialty, your general practice will have patients who will die while under hospice care, and you will want to be educated in this field as part of your commitment to a continuum of care.

Chapter 3

Chinese Culture Influences on Modern Death and Dying Issues

By comparing the history of palliative care in the US to that of China, it is possible to gain insights into the treatment of patients with Chinese medicine. China falls into the same WHO group as the US, but in a different category: countries where hospice-palliative care services are at a stage of preliminary integration into mainstream service provision. China has a long and rich cultural history which includes thousands of years of evolving Chinese medicine. China's cultural history also includes an inherent pursuit of longevity as well as shame surrounding the topics of death and dying (China Daily 2006). This has resulted in China being a latecomer to hospice care, despite the age of its medical tradition.

The search for longevity

As early as the 4th century BC, the Chinese noted that taking herbal medicine could help the sick to recover from illness. They took from this the logical conclusion that medicines could postpone death. The next step was to assume that this temporary delay might be made permanent if the right ingredients were compounded. Thus began a series of experiments (lasting over five centuries) to eradicate death by creating the "Elixir of Life" (Nieminen 2001).

The alchemical concoction results were often tragic as ingredients sometimes included extremely toxic minerals, such as lead and mercury. The search for bodily immortality cost many lives; even emperors died from elixir poisoning. Deaths from toxicity were rationalized as transformation of the physical body to an incorporeal, immortal one, but the search for the Elixir of Life lost momentum. This may be the root of the belief in traditional Chinese culture that taking medication is an aversive practice. Medications are taken for symptom relief and rarely continued past the point of obvious symptom manifestations (Wong 2007).

The traditional search for immortality incorporated preventative practices to extend longevity. In Taoism, life extension included the practice of moderation and avoidance of excess in eating, breathing, sleeping, sexual stimulation, or consuming alcohol. Herbal teas were given to reverse aging and prolong life. The focus of Traditional Chinese Medicine was prevention of illness through gentle corrections and living mindfully (Nieminen 2001).

The family

Chinese history has a continuous primary theme—a social structure with family at its center. An extended multi-generational family is considered ideal and is still common in China. In western China, in part due to restrictive reproduction ideals and modern practices, nuclear families are also common. Traditionally, the oldest adult male is the primary decision-maker. There is a long history of patriarchal and hierarchal structure in Chinese families, and a reverence for privacy regarding family matters. Conflicts regarding health and other family or personal matters are generally not discussed with non-family members (Chang and Kemp 2003).

In healthcare, including end-of-life care, the family may be the first or only providers. Finances and resources are often limited and decisions may be made based on what is best for the family (Chang and Kemp 2003). When a terminal medical diagnosis is made, it is often not disclosed to the patient. The senior relative, with other family members' input, decides how much the patient should be told.

Disclosure decisions are based on many cultural considerations. The Chinese try to protect older people from bad news. The family may withhold information or even lie to the patient. The older Chinese often believe in the Karmic law of attraction: "if you talk about bad things, you draw them to you or cause them to come true" (Wong 2007). Therefore, talking about dying is an invitation for death. Conversely, the patient may pretend that she or he does not know what is really happening.

Communications related to end-of-life issues get very complicated when the patient's prognosis is shielded. Symptom and pain management are greatly diminished when patient and family are reluctant to complain out of respect for others, particularly those in positions of authority (Chang and Kemp 2003). The relationship among family members appears to be shifting, perhaps because of the respect for elders in such situations. Absolute obedience is being replaced by greater equality and mutual respect.

There are other barriers to pain and symptom management by caregivers. These are universal, not limited to the families in China. Many people have little or no knowledge regarding the effects of pain medications or how to properly administer them. Patients often equate being a "strong" or "good" patient with postponing taking drugs, making it more difficult to control pain. Both patients and their families often fear addiction, which can lead them to withhold medication until pain becomes debilitating. Some people worry that if pain and other symptoms appear to be managed, their physicians might discount the disease's progression and fail to treat it properly.

Finally, another barrier to seeking hospice treatment is fatalism. Fatalism is the concept that events are fixed, and we are powerless to change them. In some cases, this has been a deciding factor for people to delay or refuse to seek treatment for life-limiting diseases.

After the patient dies

What happens to a person after death has been a subject of debate since the conceptualization of the human spirit. Outside the doctrines of China's multiple religions there are traditional beliefs in spirits and influences. In cities, dying patients are encouraged to go to hospitals. This practice is due to home care issues and overcrowding. It is also due in part to the belief that a death at home makes the room unusable and the house difficult to sell (Chan and Chow 2006).

Burial preparation is another family duty in many traditions. The largest religion in China is Buddhism. Buddhist families expect the oldest son or daughter to be instructed (by an older relative or person from the temple) regarding washing and dressing the body. Most Buddhists prefer burial, but after five years the physical body may be disinterred and placed in a large urn (Chang and Kemp 2003). The family decides if the urn will be reburied, or kept at home or in a temple.

For obvious reasons of diversity, it is unrealistic to generalize any culture's views on death and dying. The preceding overviews of Chinese culture and family history, although limited, are presented to help connect the past to current end-of-life care in China.

Hospice and palliative care in China

In 1987, Sontang Caring Hospital was founded in Beijing by Dr. Li Wei. Sontang was China's first hospice. Dr. Li Wei was still the hospital's medical director in 2009. There are no private beds; most patient rooms have six to eight beds. Nurses and aides also have beds in patients' rooms and live at the facility (Hospice Minnesota for Care of the Dying 2009). Hospice charges are low, but many older Chinese do not have medical insurance. Even with costs of 100 yuan (US $125) per month, and an average length stay of 31 days, many people cannot afford care. They frequently do not have pensions or their pension pay is minimal. Older people often state that they have spent too much money on their children and do not have enough for their own care (China Daily 2006).

Sontang is viewed as a good model of modern hospice care for China. People to People International Ambassador Programs bring professionals from different cultures together to learn from one another. On one such trip, a nurse with a group of 22 visiting palliative care and hospice delegates from the US noted, "We heard music playing, and no patients were crying out or appeared agitated." At Sontang, patients receive spiritual guidance in whatever religion they practice (Albright 2006). Sontang's longest recorded patient stay is five years. Its mission statement is: "To love everyone from the bottom of our hearts." In keeping with modern hospice philosophy, staff view death as a natural part of the continuum of life (Hospice Minnesota for Care of the Dying 2009).

Despite more than 32 years passing since Sontang was started, China's hospices are still rare and located only in major cities. Oncology hospitals sometimes have a few hospice wards but these are limited to fewer than 30 beds. Chinese people are still ashamed to mention death. They are just as reluctant to talk about a place to await death. Children with parents in hospices are generally seen as lacking filial piety. In most regions of China, patients prefer to die in their homes with their children beside them (China Daily 2006).

There is no federal hospice benefit in China. There is no formal home care delivery system in China. Caring for older people means that families incur expenses not covered by insurance. Compared with geriatric care, palliative care for late-stage cancer patients is more challenging due to complicated pain and symptom management. Elders in the hospices can only be tended by their family members or by non-professional nursing workers, who are mostly from rural areas (China Daily 2006).

Deficiencies in the Chinese healthcare system may become critical in the near future. China is an enormous country, with a registered population of 1.3 billion people, five times the population of the US. There is a minimum of 58 indigenous ethnic groups. Mandarin is the official language of China and is spoken by four-fifths of the population, but a number of indigenous groups speak different languages or dialects. The life expectancy is 71 years, but the healthy life expectancy is 63.2 years (Chang and Kemp 2003).

Chronic non-infectious diseases are on the rise. Eighty percent of deaths in China are due to cardiovascular disease, chronic respiratory diseases, and cancer (Strong *et al.* 2005). Regarding infectious diseases, China has the highest number of tuberculosis cases in Asia. In 2005, it was estimated that 650,000 people in China were HIV (human immunodeficiency virus) positive. In 2002, there were an estimated 130 million people in China with chronic hepatitis B and another 45 million with chronic hepatitis C. As noted above, treatment in the elderly is often delayed. This has led to an increased incidence of liver cancer resulting from hepatitis B (St. John 2002).

In larger cities, some community hospitals have a limited number of home beds, allowing patients to be attended in their homes by a small team of doctors and nurses. The large volume of non-hospice patients seen in hospitals is staggering. For instance, the Asia Pacific Community Hospital in Beijing has 460 beds and sees an additional 1000 outpatients per day. There is a shortage of registered nurses, and the number of healthcare professionals delivering home services is not sufficient for the population.

In China, medical records belong to the patients; they bring them to their appointments. The patients also make choices about tests or other procedures within the constraints of their finances (Master Travel Limited 2005). The sheer size of the population, the cultural issues, and the shortage of qualified medical professionals results in hospice care being delivered to a relatively small proportion of those in China who need it.

In-depth care for patients is limited, even when it is needed most in the terminal phase. Most palliative care services encourage patients to die at home, but it is not always possible in the cities. Many apartments have numerous family members in cramped quarters. Admitting a patient to the hospital where the best symptom management can be provided is often the most benevolent move a family can make, if they can overcome cultural beliefs and/or financial restraints. Families can still visit and talk to patients, which gives them the greatest relaxation and comfort. Despite not having hospice training, all hospital staff members consider it their duty to help care for dying patients.

Cultural attitudes, family traditions, financial limitations, emotional considerations, lack of a hospice benefit, and insufficient number of facilities have all contributed to a lack of widespread advancements in China's hospice care.

Chapter 4

East Meets West—The Face of Modern Palliative Care

Today, China and the US have strengths and weaknesses in their hospice and palliative care systems. Both countries have large populations that are uninsured and currently underserved by their healthcare systems. Both countries have nursing shortages. Both countries have too few facilities to care for their patients with life-limiting diseases. Both countries are losing the battle with preventative healthcare.

In mainland China, Traditional Chinese Medicine (TCM) is integrated with allopathic medicine to complete patient care (St. John 2002). TCM includes, but is not limited to, Chinese herbal medicine, acupuncture, qigong (slow gentle movements and breathing exercises), tui na (massage and spinal manipulation), and numerous related techniques. TCM relieves stress, reduces pain, and allows the patient to feel better. When TCM is combined with Western medicine, patients use less medication and recover more quickly from aggressive therapies (Master Travel Limited 2005).

In China, the two forms of medicine are considered complementary, not competitive. Neither school of medicine claims to be better than the other. The focus then becomes what is best for the patient. Quality of life is the goal, with no major claims towards curative intent. Overall, TCM treatments in palliative care have similar efficacy to Western treatments but tend to be gentler and have fewer side effects.

The Chinese have over 2500 years of experiential evidence that TCM works (Master Travel Limited 2005). Much of the reluctance to accept TCM in the US has come from the Western medical model of scientific double-blind experimentation. Often this focus on science disallows the holistic view of the patient which hospice philosophy tries to incorporate. Both forms of medicine use diagnosis by looking, hearing, smelling, asking, and feeling, but TCM diagnosis goes beyond signs and symptoms. It is based on a reflection of the whole individual, including, but not limited to, pulses, sounds, emotions, tongue, shen (spirit), skin, nutrition, body build, mental state, internal organs, external climate, and channels.

The US has moved forward with integrated medicine practices. By listening to their patients, oncology and palliative care practitioners are gaining greater understanding of complementary medicines and alternative therapies. Western medical treatments are covered by the insurance companies, but patients are voicing their preferences for more alternatives. Millions of dollars are spent annually on acupuncture, massage, chiropractic, and herbal treatments—and insurance companies are beginning to give discounts for preventative care practice.

What about acupuncture?

In the UK and China, acupuncture is widely integrated into palliative care settings (Leng 2013). Acupuncturists in the US have not been able to duplicate this effort yet. Our profession is titled as certified or licensed acupuncturists (in the majority of states). Often people think of acupuncturists on the same par as massage therapists. There is a failure to recognize the distinction between a technique or therapy and a comprehensive, energetic healthcare system. Equally, the public has a general lack of understanding of the educational requirements, degrees, or the number of hours needed to become a practitioner. It is essential to expand the public view of us as practitioners of Asian Medicine, and recognize that the minimum 3 year (1905 hours) Master's degree and completion of the national board certification is on the same level as nurse practitioners or physicians' assistants.

Asian Medicine, much like hospice, embraces a whole-person pattern approach of mind, body, and spirit. It is unique in that the system utilizes a multitude of therapies including (but not limited to) acupuncture, Asian bodywork (e.g. shiatsu, acupressure, tui na), Chinese herbal medicines, cupping, coining, electrostimulation, heat therapies, meditation, moxibustion, nutrition, qigong, and tai chi. Most of these therapies may be useful in terminal disease treatments, though there may be some contraindications depending on the individual patient's condition. In particular, acupuncture, using specific point combinations, can serve to calm and release emotional and spiritual concerns for hospice patients (McPhail *et al.* 2018).

Many hospice patients experience physical discomfort along with the emotional reality of the dying process. Acupuncture is a safe and inexpensive treatment for physical conditions that are common among hospice and palliative care patients. Many Asian Medicine randomized controlled trials in the UK and the US have been limited to acupuncture as the sole modality. In one group of studies, acupuncture was found to be useful for treating nausea, vomiting, dyspnea (shortness of breath), and, most importantly, pain, in a drug-free way, without side effects (Kaufman and Salkeld 2008). Non-painful symptoms such as dyspnea, hot flushes, xerostomia, and a variety of radiation-induced side effects, including bladder and bowel problems, and radionecrotic ulcers, have had variable, but generally positive outcomes when treated with acupuncture (Filshie and Rubens 2011).

Like most of the therapies listed in the interdisciplinary team outline, acupuncture aims at patient relaxation and improving quality of life. Acupuncture can powerfully reduce physical, mental and emotional distress. It can help a person tap into their spiritual resources when they need them the most. Acupuncture points that act at the spirit level are extremely therapeutic. Whether by reducing fear and spiritual suffering or activating elemental functions that ease dying, acupuncture can help patients accept the inevitable, and to die peacefully. The dying patient gains a greater sense of peace and a stronger connection to the subtle energies of their deeper spiritual essence. They are able to honestly accept the dissolution of the body and their physical existence.

The World Health Organization (WHO) recognizes acupuncture as an adjunctive therapy for palliative care patients, and some studies have recommended it for insurance reimbursement in end-of-life care. The WHO has approved acupuncture for many other conditions found in end-of-life patients, including: cardiovascular, dermatological, eye/ear/throat-related, gynecological/obstetric, musculoskeletal, neurological, psychological/emotional, and respiratory symptoms (Melbourne Zen Hospice 2009).

Research and cost effectiveness

A great deal of time and money has been spent on cancer research, and though it is beyond the scope of this manual to discuss oncology, some interesting research related to palliative care is worth noting.

Heart disease and cancer are the leading causes of death in the US and the UK. After being diagnosed with cancer, more than 70 percent of patients will use some form of complementary and alternative medicine (CAM), and 16 percent will see a CAM provider (Lafferty et al. 2008). National healthcare costs for CAM in the US have been difficult to track due to practitioners with cash-only practices and lack of insurance coverage.

Washington State passed legislation in 1996 that required every category of licensed healthcare provider to be covered by private insurance. The mandate included acupuncturists turning their treatments into commercial insurance products and creating a large bank of insurance claims data. The following information was the result of a study on cancer patients in Washington from 2000 to 2004 (Lafferty et al. 2008). The predominant forms of insurance coverage were point-of-service plans, preferred provider organizations, and group policies.

Of the 900,000 patient files reviewed, only 2900 met criteria for the study. Patients were aged from 18 to 64 and had diagnoses of breast, colorectal, hematologic, lung, or prostate cancer. Caucasian women with an average age of 54 and a diagnosis of breast cancer were the largest single group to use CAM. Out of all the patients, 26.5 percent used some form of CAM (including acupuncturists, chiropractors, massage therapists, and naturopathic physicians). Musculoskeletal issues were the most common diagnoses made by conventional and CAM providers, including almost 70 percent of all acupuncture visits.

Acupuncture was used by 1.3 percent of the population of the study. Of 895 patients receiving chemotherapy, 50 percent had a diagnosis of nausea and vomiting, but only 26 of these patients (5.7%) visited an acupuncturist. In the 12 months preceding death, the median number of patient visits to CAM providers was two. Close to 58 percent of the patients who died used hospice care at the end of life. Expenditures for CAM treatments were significantly lower than costs for conventional providers throughout the entire study. It is interesting to note that from 2005, in Washington, 86 percent of hospices offered massage to their patients, but acupuncture was only offered by 32 percent.

Growth potential for hospice and palliative care

For some advanced diseases, there simply is no cure. In these cases, continuing treatments is costly and ineffective and sometimes detrimental to the patient's already compromised health. At this time, palliative care, with a focus on symptom management and comfort, may improve the quality of life for the patient's remaining time.

In 1978, the US Department of Health, Education, and Welfare published a report on hospice. They welcomed the hospice model as a reduced-cost care option for terminally ill patients. Medicare coverage followed, allowing hospices to grow from grassroots, mostly volunteer-run organizations into large healthcare companies. There are more than 4382 hospices today, with different working models— some are independent, others are non-profit agencies. For-profit hospice companies are often part of hospitals or health systems (Hospice of Michigan 2009).

In 1999, one in four Americans at the end of life (approximately 700,000) received hospice care (National Hospice and Palliative Care Organization 2009b). That is close to the same percentage of people in the US who have written instructions for their end-of-life care. Despite the fact that it has been five decades since Elisabeth Kübler-Ross wrote *On Death and Dying* (1969), Americans are very reluctant to talk to their aging parents about end-of-life decisions. Research shows that parents are more willing to talk with their children about safe sex and drugs than about their own end-of-life decisions.

In 2019, according to the National Hospice and Palliative Care Organization, its population is grossly underserved. It estimates that only one in three patients who could benefit from hospice services are actually receiving care.

Who pays for hospice?

Under the Medicare Hospice Benefit, Americans who are terminally ill are guaranteed (at little or no cost) comprehensive, high-quality end-of-life care. This is extended to Medicare beneficiaries and their families. After a physician certifies that a patient has a life expectancy of six months or less, their case is reviewed for the first two 90-day periods of care. If the patient is still alive after these six months, their case is reviewed every 60 days. There is no limit to the number of 60-day reviews, as long as their physician still certifies that they have a life-limiting prognosis.

Most hospices have a large volunteer component, supported by their local communities. Hospices can receive grants, and funds from foundations, and many have ongoing fundraising events. Hospice care is sometimes incorporated with home health agencies or hospitals—often with a separate building. Payments from Medicaid and private health insurance are also forms of patient care reimbursement. However, the US hospice benefits are funded under Medicare, part A, and if left unchanged, that fund is expected to run out in 2026, leaving millions without hospital or hospice coverage.

Financial planning for long-term disability is an important and often omitted topic of discussion. In the US, most hospice services (90%) are provided in the home, so it is important to know what medications, treatments, and equipment are covered.

Family members serve as the main hands-on caregivers, and ties can be strained if the family has to pay for uncovered expenses. For insurance purposes, "care" is defined by the setting in which services are delivered. Patients and their families need to know well before hospice or palliative care is needed whether insurance or some other payor will cover it.

Who regulates hospices?

There are federal regulations and standards of compliance that each hospice must meet in order to be approved for Medicare reimbursement. Hospices that are Medicare-certified must provide nursing, pharmacy, and doctor services around the clock. Licensing requirements vary from state to state. Each state has standards that must be met for hospice care. In order to ensure quality care, the National Hospice and Palliative Care Organization (2009a) has written recommendations in its publication entitled *Standards of Practice for Hospice Programs*. There are accreditation organizations that evaluate hospice programs to protect consumers. Many hospice programs volunteer to obtain accreditation.

How does hospice work?

In an ideal world, the patient and family have discussed the disease process and care options for their given situation long before it becomes a pressing concern. Such conversations can greatly reduce stress and allow the patient to have autonomy in the decision-making process. In reality, this does not always happen, and the patient may feel that the family is giving up. Often, hospice care is not started soon enough, and the patient may be suffering with poorly controlled symptoms. Ideally, the patient, their family, and the doctor will decide together when hospice care should begin. (American Cancer Society 2009)

The patient's doctor will determine if the patient meets criteria for hospice care, and will make a formal request or a "referral" for such. A member of the hospice interdisciplinary team (usually an intake nurse, nurse case manager, and/or a social worker) will make an effort to visit the patient within 48 hours of that referral. If the patient's situation is considered urgent, services may begin sooner.

The Palliative Performance Scale

In 1996, a group of people working with the Victoria Hospice in British Columbia, created the Palliative Performance Scale (PPS) as a means to paint a general picture of a patient's health, or decline. Each hospice patient is assigned a performance level (expressed as a percentage of 100, by 10s, i.e. 100% is totally health, 0% is dead). The score is based on the ability to walk, to work or participate in a regular daily schedule of events, signs of physical or mental disease-based decline, and the patient's ability to eat or drink and to be awake and aware or responsive to people, places, and things (Anderson *et al.* 1996). The score a patient is initially given and overall changes in condition can affect payments and the level of care they may receive. At hospice interdisciplinary team meetings, the staff provides input (based on their observations and patient/caregiver reporting), to assure the percentage level is correct.

This interdisciplinary healthcare team manages hospice care, and someone is on call 24 hours a day, 7 days a week. A full-time registered nurse generally provides care for about a dozen patients. Social workers may see two to three times the number of patients/families as nurses. In most cases, patient visits by nurses are required at least once every two weeks, but often hospices prefer patients to be seen twice a week. Home health aides provide personal care to the patient and may be scheduled for visits anywhere from one to five times a week. The nurse provides a plan of care, and all visits are based on the patient and family needs, as well as the condition of the patient during the course of illness.

Hospice care relies heavily on volunteers. They provide many different types of support to patients and their loved ones, including social interaction, emotional comfort, and companionship. Volunteers sometimes stay with a patient to give caregivers a break, or run errands, and prepare light meals if the family is reluctant to leave the patient.

As noted earlier, most hospice care happens at home, but it can also be managed in an assisted living facility, a nursing home (or long-term care center), a hospital, or a private hospice facility. A patient may also go into a facility for respite care, often up to five days, to give the caretaker a break. If the patient is placed in a nursing home, there will be a written agreement in place in order for the hospice to serve residents of the facility. The patient may only need short-term skilled care and can return home when they and their caregiver are ready.

Patient and caregiver education about the dying process is also offered by the staff. The team manages all aspects of transfers (from home to facilities or facility to facility) and deaths. Usually, a hospice nurse and social worker will be responsible for interacting with the family, home care agency or inpatient facility staff, the medical equipment and supply companies, the doctor, and other community professionals, such as pharmacists, clergy, coroner, and funeral directors.

Hospice services do not end at death. Bereavement services are usually offered to surviving loved ones. Support for mourning in their time of loss is provided via phone calls, visits, cards, or letters—and is offered as an ongoing service for a year in most hospice models. A professional social worker, counselor, clergy member, or a specially trained volunteer may provide these services. Some hospices may have ongoing bereavement support groups or may direct people to community groups, if available.

Why hospice, why now?

According to the United States Census Bureau (2019), the US population is estimated to be over 329.6 million. Of 2.8 million Americans who died in 2016 (over 2 million died from chronic and debilitating diseases (Centers for Disease Control and Prevention 2017)), fewer than 25 percent actually died at home. When polled, however, 80 percent of Americans stated they wished to die at home. There is a disconnect between the general population and hospice information. Americans want these types of services, but 83 percent of them don't know about the scope of hospice care. When informed, 66 percent of patients needing end-of-life care stated they would welcome help from an outside organization like a hospice.

Of the 1.43 million patients served by hospice care each year, 75 percent were able to die in the comfort of their own home. Due to population constraints, these services cannot be expected to be handled by the current healthcare system. There were 4382 Medicare certified hospices operating in the US in 2017 (National Hospice and Palliative Care Organization 2017).

The average annual expenditure on healthcare increases annually. Baby boomers have emphasized living well. Indeed, according to the latest statistics, they are the last American generation expected to live longer than their parents' generation. Living well also means dying well, and the discussions taking place in the media, online, and in other arenas confirm this ideal.

On March 28, 2016, the worldwide number of people over 65 years of age was 617 million. In 2006, the oldest baby boomers (born between 1946 and 1964) began turning 60 years old, and it is estimated there will be 1.6 billion people over 65 in 2050. The people needing and expecting hospice services in the next 30 years will be one of the largest, most influential groups of people in the history of the world.

Listed below are statistics from 2016 on deaths worldwide. Please note that most of the top ten causes for death are disease processes where the patient could be sick for a prolonged period and would be considered appropriate for hospice care.

- Cardiovascular diseases 17.65 million

- Cancers 8.93 million

- Respiratory disease 3.54 million

- Diabetes, blood and endocrine disease 3.19 million

- Lower respiratory infections 2.57 million

- Dementia 2.38 million

- Neonatal deaths 1.73 million

- Diarrheal diseases 1.66 million

- Road incidents 1.34 million

- Liver disease 1.26 million

- Tuberculosis 1.21 million

- Kidney disease 1.19 million

- Digestive disease 1.09 million

- HIV/AIDS 1.03 million

- Suicide 817,148

- Malaria 719,551

- Homicide 390,794

- Nutritional deficiencies 368,107

- Drowning 302,932

- Meningitis 295,879

- Protein-energy malnutrition 236,430

- Maternal deaths 230,615

- Parkinson's disease 211,296

- Alcohol disorder 173,893

- Intestinal infectious diseases 155,449

- Drug disorders 143,775

- Hepatitis 134,045

- Fire 132,084

- Conflict 115,782

- Heat-related deaths (hot or cold exposure) 55,596

- Terrorism 34,676

- Natural disasters 7059.

Adapted from Ritchie and Roger 2019

In short, there is a huge market in a field of medicine that embraces holistic care for Asian Medicine practitioners who have the sensitivity and creativity to help terminally ill patients. To put it simply, everyone dies. Palliative care patients have some time to process options and choose treatments that fit their perception of what it should feel like to be cared for. The picture is missing one thing—YOU!

Part of our job as practitioners is educating the general public, patients, and other healthcare professionals. There is a national trend to integrate medicine, but we must be careful not to dilute the potency of Asian Medicine. Inform everyone to ask practitioners about their education, and explain the levels of training each professional category requires in order to ensure they receive the most professional acupuncture care available for optimum health and wellness. Acupuncture should only be administered by practitioners who have specific education in this field. Teach your patients that inadequate understanding of Oriental medical diagnostic procedures can lead to energy imbalances and improper needling techniques that can lead to health risks or diminished results (Council of Colleges of Acupuncture and Oriental Medicine 2009).

The interdisciplinary team

In the US, an interdisciplinary healthcare team manages hospice care. The traditional hospice interdisciplinary team is made up of many interacting disciplines, with a core of Western medical roles. Hospice staff members are trained to assess and treat physical discomfort and emotional and spiritual distress. This core group meets on a regular basis to assess patient care and progress.

The hospice team empowers patients and families to manage difficult situations and to foster spiritual and personal growth. Team members receive special training which helps them to effectively anticipate disease-related symptoms and to use preventative interventions to ease pain, manage side effects, and prepare the patients and their families for the death and dying process. Family conferences are scheduled with team members to make certain everyone has a clear picture of the patient's needs and current condition.

Irene Harrison (2008) compiled some of the roles involved in interdisciplinary teams, of whose duties are described and expanded upon here:

- *The medical director* is a physician who provides expertise in hospice care to the interdisciplinary team. They attend team meetings and review feedback from team members to guide the staff in providing appropriate care for the terminally ill. The medical director consults with the patient's primary care physician and educates other doctors regarding the philosophy and practice of hospice medicine.

- *Social workers* focus on the emotional and social needs of patients and their family members or caregivers. They offer problem-solving skills and links to community services, advocating for patients and facilitating communication between involved parties with sensitivity to cultural and social diversity. If the family is not living close to a patient, the social worker may call with updates on the patient's condition. They encourage the patient and family members to share feelings in conferences or informally on a daily basis.

- *Hospice nurses* are the key to effective pain and symptom management. They work as case managers and see patients in their primary living situations. Nurses provide highly skilled, coordinated care and communicate with family members or other caregivers to assure patient comfort.

- *Home health aides* provide hands-on personal care tasks like bathing, feeding, peri-anal hygiene, and grooming for terminally ill patients. Due to these intimate tasks, and the amount of time such care requires, patients often confide in and feel more comfortable with home health aides than with other team members. Aides are a vital link in assuring proper care. They communicate with nurses, reporting any noted changes in the patient's physical condition or emotional state.

- *Chaplains* help patients to get in touch with their religious or spiritual beliefs. Patients with life-limiting illnesses often search for the existential meaning of their lives. The chaplain tends to the patients' spiritual needs by allowing them to review and explore their values, beliefs, and fears about life and what happens after dying. A patient may have their own clerical support or be referred to community support if the team does not have a chaplain.

- *The pharmacist* uses working knowledge of medication effects, potencies, and interactions to maximize pain control and symptom relief while minimizing side effects.

Additional members

Not all team members come to meetings, and any of the following may be asked to attend a family conference, or may be called in for special consultations and treatments:

- *Nutritionists* monitor the patient's eating habits, including appetite and taste changes and weight losses or gains. They can be of special help to families, who get particularly upset when their loved ones eat minimally or stop taking food or fluid by mouth. The nutritionist knows the natural progression of terminal illnesses, and can help families or caregivers alleviate their worries that the patient will die of starvation.

- *Volunteers* are essential unpaid workers in most hospice programs. Volunteer services range from hands-on patient care to office work or fundraising for the hospice. Volunteers require training prior to working with patients. They are taught the philosophy, history, and details of hospice care. They should understand the supporting and facilitating roles of the hospice interdisciplinary team members, and know basic principles of pain and symptom management for the patient. Volunteers learn the physical, social, emotional, and spiritual needs of the terminally ill patients and their families. They discuss and experience loss and grief in hospice patients, families, volunteers, and staff members, and they are encouraged to explore their own values and philosophy in relation to life and death (Schwartz 2009).

- *Physical therapists* help the patient to maintain their range of motion and ability to get in and out of bed, use chairs, and access transportation. They assess the patient for self-care abilities, including feeding, grooming, and bathing capabilities. They evaluate the patient for functional changes and suggest modifications as needed to maintain patient safety.

- *Occupational therapists* help patients adapt to living conditions or environments to conserve their energy in order to perform the activities of daily living with the highest level of independence. Their interventions purposefully promote health and prevent injuries.

- *Speech and language pathologists* assess patients' speech, language, swallowing, and cognitive aspects of communication, and also their sensory awareness related to these abilities. In patients where these abilities have been compromised, pathologists work to develop alternate communication systems. When swallowing is an issue, they coordinate with team members to help patients meet their nutritional needs.

- *Psychologists or psychiatrists* may be consulted on difficult cases. Depression is a common problem with patients near the end of life, and other pre-existing psychological problems often require special interventions or medication adjustments.

The variety of skills and expertise of the interdisciplinary team accentuate the special care patients and their families need as they near the end of life.

Other therapies offered by modern hospices

At this point, you may find yourself asking, "Where are the acupuncturists?" Along with the above interdisciplinary team members, hospices may employ the following additional therapies as part of the services they offer:

- *Animal therapy* uses dogs, horses (including miniature horses), cats, monkeys, rabbits, birds, or other animals that interact with patients. Patients focus on animals as part of symptom management and/or grief support. A therapy team is usually made up of a specially trained animal, its owner, and a hospice social worker.

- *Aromatherapy*, also known as essential oil therapy, uses active and passive inhalation of extracts from plants to help relieve physical and emotional conditions. This is a safe and effective therapy with no side effects and can be used to treat physical symptoms such as pain and nausea, as well as emotional symptoms, including depression and anxiety.

- *Art therapy* incorporates art and craft materials for drawing and other art projects in conjunction with psychotherapy. People choose a particular medium, such as clay or collage, to create art that aids or expresses the mind, body, and spirit.

- *Creative or expressive arts therapies* use art, movement, dance, writing, and other creative tools for expressing and examining feelings, body issues, emotions, and thoughts.

- *Energy medicine* in this case refers to therapies based on the concept of qi (also spelled chi or ki, and pronounced "chee"), commonly accepted in Western culture to be the flow of energy that sustains human beings. Energy medicine includes, but is in no way limited to, acupuncture, Reiki, qigong, therapeutic touch, intercessory prayer, and shiatsu. These have their roots in ancient medicine. The common belief of all these medicines is that physical and emotional illnesses are a result of the imbalances in the natural flow of qi in the body, and that energy medicine can restore balance to optimize health.

- *Hypnotherapy* is a focused state of awareness applied to modify the patient's emotions, behaviors, and attitudes. Hypnotherapy can help hospice patients by reducing pain, nausea and vomiting, anxiety and stress-related illnesses, including depression, and spiritual suffering. Through subconscious suggestions, hypnotherapy can promote feelings of well-being leading to increased relaxation and better sleep patterns.

- *Massage therapy* is the practice of manipulating soft tissues (including skin and muscles) with physical, functional, and psychological purpose. It is practiced to promote relaxation of the body and support its ability to heal itself.

- *Music thanatology* focuses on the use of music vigils to help the dying patient and others present relax into a meditative state. A prescription for comfort care is composed of voice and harp music. Often, after a music vigil, the patient is less agitated, has diminished pain and decreased respiratory distress, and experiences more restorative sleep. The healing power of music often aids in the resolution of spiritual, familial, and emotional issues.

Adapted from Denver Hospice 2009

Chapter 5

Integrating Acupuncture into Current Hospice and Palliative Care Models

L et's go further and look deeper into the world of hospice care
  and palliative medicine.

How do we build a bridge without being swept down the river? We have already started the process. More allopathic models are including Asian Medicine in the treatment of hospice and palliative care patients. As an acupuncturist, you must realize that you speak a foreign language. When you start talking to a patient about liver qi stagnation, their eyes usually glaze over, and they end up going home telling their loved ones, "There is something wrong with my liver."

The same holds true for doctors, nurses, social workers, and other allied professionals. When you speak using the same terminology to a doctor, you are mostly going to hear them say, "There is no such thing," or "That is not the Western medicine function of the liver." And, of course, there is no ICD-10 code[1] for liver qi stagnation. You are a stranger in a strange land. To communicate effectively, you must speak the language.

---

1 The World Health Organization created a medical classification list, the International Statistical Classification of Diseases and Related Health Problems (ICD). The tenth revision of this list, ICD-10, is used in medical coding and billing.

In order for our patients to understand the value of our medicine, they must have it explained to them in terms that don't leave them overwhelmed with information, or unable to comprehend the process. We know that as soon as the mind comes across an idea or statement it does not understand, further conversation or information is much more likely to be lost. The logical part of the brain will still be stuck trying to create, or problem solve, the concept, or define the term for which it has no prior knowledge.

In order for allopathic medical practitioners to understand the value of Asian Medicine, we must talk to them in their own language. A combination of randomized controlled trials, research studies, and medical terminology will work the best to communicate your message.

In order for insurance companies to understand the value of Asian Medicine, we must also learn to speak in terms of the positive consequences of preventative medicine. Help them to grasp the financial savings of acupuncture over other treatments. Relate decreased potential liability to limited side effects or negative reactions. The bottom line is that we want to be a part of the complete medical team in order to give the best patient care, and we deserve to be paid for it.

As acupuncturists, we need to remain focused on patient care that leaves the patient feeling supported and allows them to use their voice. We do not let our patient time be diluted by others. Building a bridge with the allopathic model does not mean that we allow our treatment times to be put in a fast lane. We foster an environment of mutual respect by educating other practitioners about our standard of care, including the duration and frequency of treatment sessions.

How do we accomplish this? We practice excellent communication. Start with the basics. Consider this is a primer. Think of the questions that you are asked most frequently regarding acupuncture. We must be prepared to answer these questions in simple language for patients, and in scientific terms for medical specialists. The following could be used as a guide for giving a five-minute lecture to your local hospice interdisciplinary team(s).

What does acupuncture do, or how does it work?

Over the years, there have been many explanations about what acupuncture does. Each point has functions and indications; for instance, for the point LI 14 (Binao), the functions are to open the nasal passages and to disperse wind heat conditions. The symptoms it is indicated for are rhinitis, nosebleeds, and round worms in the abdomen. This is not a scientific explanation of how it works, it is an experiential explanation based on observations of the use of the point, and results experienced by hundreds of thousands of patients. That does not make it any less valid, but the current allopathic model requires scientifically verifiable proof and repeatable results.

For five thousand years, we did not have the instrumentation or technology to see the meridians or measure qi. Remember, it wasn't that long ago in human history that we could not see protozoa, then Van Leeuwenhoek improved the microscope which opened the door to the science of microbiology. Practical electrocardiograms weren't invented until 1903, and the EEGs, which are now used every day, were developed in 1924. They helped us to measure the electroconductivity of the heart and brain, and we believed that acupuncture worked via neural energy.

As technology advances, we are learning ways to measure the effects of acupuncture along the meridians, or the pathways associated with the organs. New groundbreaking research shows that the insertion of an acupuncture needle into the skin disrupts the branching point of nerves called C fibers. These C fibers transmit low-grade sensory information over very long distances by using Merkel cells as intermediaries. Dr. Morry Silberstein of the Curtin University of Technology has completed his research, which specifically pinpoints that the C fibers actually branch exactly at acupuncture points.

Scientists are uncertain what role C fibers play in the nervous system, but Dr. Silverstein theorizes that the bundle of nerves exists to maintain arousal or wakefulness. The insertion of the acupuncture needle disrupts this circuit and numbs our sensitivity to pain. He goes on to say that acupuncture points show lower electrical resistance than other nearby areas of the skin. Which means these are points of greater conductivity. Dr. Silverstein's research is available in the *Journal of Theoretical Biology* (Vlasto 2018). He states:

> In the absence of a scientific rationale, acupuncture has not been widely used in the mainstream medical community. If we can explain the process scientifically, we can open it to full scientific scrutiny and develop ways to use it as a part of medical treatments.

Acupuncture for pain relief is actually being taught to American Air Force physicians by Dr. Richard Niemtzow, a consultant for complementary and alternative medicine for the Surgeon General of the Air Force. He created a technique called "Battlefield Acupuncture," which relieves severe pain for several days. It utilizes very tiny semi-permanent needles at specific acupoints on the skin of the ear that block pain signals from reaching the brain. He has stated, "This is one of the fastest pain attenuators in existence. The pain can be gone in five minutes" (Vlasto 2018).

A North Korean researcher, Kim Bonghan, published papers in the early 1960s and his research was confirmed by the Japanese researchers Fujiwara and Yu in 1967 (Soh 2004). Unfortunately, his research took almost 40 years to be confirmed through studies done on rats, rabbits, and pigs with stereo-microscope photographs and electron microscopy. The images of acupuncture meridians are assemblies of tubular structures 30–100 micro-meters wide (red blood cells are 6–8 micro-meters in diameter).

These structures have remained undiscovered for so long because they are almost transparent and so thin that they are barely visible with low-magnification surgical microscopes. They are also easily confused with fibrin, which coagulates and obscures these structures when there is bleeding in dissected tissues. Now that they have been rediscovered, researchers are investigating their composition and function. The tubular structures that make up Bonghan channels contain a flowing liquid that includes abundant hyaluronic acid, a substance that cushions and lubricates the joints, eyes, skin, and even heart valves.

Small granules of DNA or micro-cells about 1–2 micro-meters in diameter that contain chromosomal material highly reactive to stem cell antibody stains were also visible in the stereo-microscope photographs. When these cells were isolated and then induced to differentiate, they grew into cells of all three germ layers. Bonghan states, "These may be our body's natural source of pluripotent adult stem cells, with the potential to develop into any cell in the body" (Vlasto 2018).

Russian researchers in 1991 at the Institute for Clinical and Experimental Medicine in Novosibirsk (Vlasto 2018), in a research project lasting several years, discovered how the human body conducts light. They found that the light-conducting ability of the human body exists only along the meridians, and can enter and exit only along the acupuncture points.

Dr. Kaznachejew, a professor of physics, was quoted as saying:

> This seems to prove that we have a light transferral system in our body somewhat like optical fiber. It appears that the light can even travel when the light canal is bent, or totally twisted. The light appears to be reflected from the inner surface, appearing to go in some sort of zigzag track. You can explain this through traditional electromagnetic light theory as it is used in optical fiber communications. (Vlasto 2018)

This finding has been confirmed by a 1992 study in the *Journal of Traditional Chinese Medicine* and a 2005 study in the *Journal of Alternative and Complementary Medicine* where moxibustion and infrared thermography were used to trace meridian pathways (Vlasto 2018).

For presentation purposes, you can summarize the above reports by stating that scientific research has revealed that the acupuncture points are places where C fibers branch, and by inserting needles into these points it creates a long-lasting stimulation of the nervous system. The meridians these points lie on are made of Bonghan channels, which contain hyaluric acid (to lubricate the joints, eyes, skin, and heart valves) and pluripotent adult stem cells (which can develop into any cell in the body).

Does it hurt?

Patients who have undergone blood tests, IVs (intravenous therapy/ fluids), and subcutaneous or intramuscular injections can develop fear of needles. It is important to explain to your patients that acupuncture needles are not beveled to cut the skin, nor are they hollow to inject fluids. Often, the pain from a shot is from the pressure of fluid being injected under the skin, into a muscle, or into the vein. There are exceptions—some of the nine classic needles can inflict pain, and there are acupuncturists who are currently using injection therapies which require a hollow-form needle.

For some people, after an acupuncture needle is placed there is a sensation of warmth or tingling. This effect is known as "de qi," when healing energy arrives at the needle. Other people experience a feeling of numbness, or simply feel nothing at all. Usually these sensations give way to a greater sense of calmness and relaxation. Being hydrated is one way to assure less pain.

How many needles do you use?

In hospice and palliative care, we use as few needles as possible. In some cases, if the patient is very weak or frail, or bruises too easily, we may use gentle finger pressure on the points, or magnets, seeds, or energetic treatments if contact cannot be tolerated.

How many treatments does it require to be effective?

Each person has their own timing and specific needs. As a general rule, acute disorders require a shorter course of treatments than chronic disorders. Depending on the duration, severity, and nature of the patient's illness, they may need a single treatment or require a series of 2–15, or more. Often patients come under hospice care with little time left to live, so you may only get the chance to do one or two treatments. Again, the goal in hospice treatments is any possible symptom relief, and, more importantly, emotional comfort leading to a peaceful acceptance of death as the natural end of a life cycle.

Does insurance cover it, or how do you get paid for treatments?

In some states, acupuncture is covered under Medicaid. Private insurance plans may cover acupuncture, but often limit the number of visits a person can have in a year. Many hospices fund patient treatments from various gifts, grants, or funds that they have allocated for complementary or alternative treatments, or miscellaneous expenses. Currently, Medicare is not covering acupuncture treatments; however, this year Medicare is paying for some acupuncture research on patients with lower back pain. On a positive note, the Veterans Administration hospitals use acupuncture for pain, substance abuse, including opioid addiction, and post-traumatic stress disorder. This new trend to cover treatments with federal funding gives credence to the idea that acupuncture may be covered under Medicare in the foreseeable future. Healthcare in the US has fallen behind many other countries where acupuncture is covered under universal medical coverage.

What can you use acupuncture for in palliative care?

Before answering this question, let's take a closer look at the broader concept of palliative care.

Palliative care is focused on symptom relief. It is not meant to be curative, but instead, the primary goal is to improve the patient's quality of life through symptom management and control. Palliative care patients may have a disease that is serious and currently incurable. The disease may be life-limiting, but may be slow moving in its process, so the patient's condition is not terminal. For instance, a person who has the early stages of chronic obstructive pulmonary disease, or Parkinsonism, may need palliative care. The primary problem is the amazingly large chasm between patients who are still able-bodied and those who are eligible for, or in need of, skilled nursing services.

Palliative care in the US is based on a need for skilled nursing care. The way the current healthcare model treats people who have a disease but no manageable symptoms is to monitor them until they do. There is little proactive or preventative medicine for subclinical signs and symptoms. Acupuncture could be working to arrest or reverse patterns of disharmony, to give these patients a better quality of life, but without insurance coverage, we are limited to providing care to those who can afford to pay cash, or to offering discounted or free treatments. These limits often dilute the potential for Asian Medicine to be delivered at its optimum level and to achieve maximum patient benefits.

Palliative care does provide for patients' needs such as oxygen use and education, wound care, emotional care, and other therapies delivered by skilled professionals that are covered by general health insurance. The truth of the matter is that these criteria have changed over the years, and in the US, hospice and palliative care insurance coverage is subject to federal, and state, variations.

Hospice care by its nature and approach is palliative, but it is distinguished by the fact that it is for terminally ill patients. How do we know when a person is going to die? The simple answer is, we don't. Predicting the exact date or hour of a person's death is in the same category as predicting the date or hour of a person's birth—it is based on factual knowledge, and sprinkled with a best guess. The physician gathers information that leads them to define someone as being terminally ill. The physician's opinion is based on the formula that "the 'normal' person, under 'normal' circumstances, will follow a 'standard' disease progression, and die within the next six-month period."

The exception to determining when a person is going to die is when they enter a stage of decline called "active dying." There are physical signs and stressors that make it easier to say that they have less than a week, or less than a day. In the end, these are still the best guesses of the caregivers, as patients have been known to rally or, conversely, die with great brevity.

This six-month timeline in America is really fueled by the insurance industry's rigid standards. These rules are in place to prevent fraud, which is understandable, but they can also lead to negative consequences. The patient is initially certified by their physician or the hospice medical director for 90 days, and must be re-certified for a second 90-day period. If the patient is still alive at the end of the initial six-month period, the requirement changes and the physician must then re-certify the patient every 60 days, signing a form that states that the patient is terminally ill with a life expectancy of six months or less if the terminal illness runs its normal course.

The requirement for the hospice team to prove the patient is eligible for re-certification has led to an unnatural focus on patient decline. Team members are schooled to write notes geared to assure hospice insurance coverage. It has led to computerized charting at the bedside, with extremely long and repetitive forms for hospice nurses, social workers, and chaplains. Completing these forms often causes unnecessary fatigue for the patient. Unfortunately, the requirements to prove patient decline have swung too far. In some instances, they are so strict they have led to patients being discharged prematurely from hospice, leaving them to die without proper care.

Just to be clear, the Centers for Medicare and Medicaid Services (CMS) defines "terminal illness" as: "An individual is considered to be terminally ill if the medical prognosis is that the individual's life expectancy is 6 months or less if the illness runs its normal course" (Department of Health and Human Services 2018).

Of course, a running subtext in hospice care is that there really isn't any such thing as a "normal" patient. There are always patients who die unexpectedly, or live much longer than what seems humanly possible. These cases aren't probable, and yet they still fall within the range of the possible normal outcomes for hospice care.

In 2016, in the US, 1.43 million Medicare participants were enrolled in hospice for one day or more. 1.04 million Medicare beneficiaries died while enrolled in hospice care in 2016. The average length of service for a person under Medicare in a hospice was 71 days, and that included people who had been enrolled from the previous year and were still under care, and people who had been discharged from hospice care but were later readmitted. The median length of service was 24 days. That means 715,000 patients were in hospice care for 24 days or fewer before they most likely died or were discharged (National Hospice and Palliative Care Organization 2017). The bottom line here is that this is a very short time to prepare to die—mentally, physically, spiritually, or financially.

Now, let's ask that most important question again.

What can you use acupuncture for in hospice and palliative care?

Many practitioners start their practices with literature that includes the World Health Organization list. It is an extensive, generalized list meant to impress patients with the variety of conditions that acupuncture can treat. The list is based on a prestigious cataloging of information about randomized controlled trials, studies, compilations, and other papers on the effects of acupuncture and Asian medical treatments.

The World Health Organization (WHO) (2003) has listed the following symptoms, diseases, and conditions that have been shown through controlled trials to be treated effectively by acupuncture:

- Low back pain

- Neck pain

- Sciatica

- Tennis elbow

- Knee pain

- Periarthritis of the shoulder

- Sprains

- Facial pain (including craniomandibular disorders)

- Headache

- Dental pain

- Temporomandibular (TMJ) dysfunction

- Rheumatoid arthritis

- Induction of labor

- Correction of malposition of fetus (breech presentation)

- Morning sickness

- Nausea and vomiting

- Postoperative pain

- Stroke

- Essential hypertension

- Primary hypotension

- Renal colic

- Leucopenia

- Adverse reactions to radiation or chemotherapy

- Allergic rhinitis, including hay fever

- Biliary colic

- Depression (including depressive neurosis and depression following stroke)

- Acute bacillary dysentery

- Primary dysmenorrhea

- Acute epigastralgia

- Peptic ulcer

- Acute and chronic gastritis.

The list is long, quite old (it was published originally in 1998), and fairly general. It contains medical terms unfamiliar to many patients—words like leucopenia, bacillary dysentery, dysmenorrhea, and epigastralgia—so it might be best to present it when educating medical professions.

There are three further classifications from the WHO:

- Diseases, symptoms, and conditions for which the therapeutic effect of acupuncture has been shown, but further proof is needed.

- Diseases, symptoms, and conditions for which the therapeutic effect of acupuncture is worth trying.

- Diseases, symptoms, and conditions for which acupuncture may be tried, provided the practitioner has special modern medical knowledge and adequate monitoring equipment. These include more specific life-limiting conditions such as:

   - breathlessness in chronic obstructive pulmonary disease

- coma

- coronary heart disease (angina pectoris)

- paralysis, progressive bulbar, and pseudobulbar.

One study (Romeo *et al.* 2015) looked at acupuncture to treat generalized symptoms of patients in a palliative care setting. Twenty-six patients participated in an acupuncture trial, receiving a course of weekly treatments that ranged from 1 to 14 weeks. The average number of treatments was five. The Edmonton Symptom Assessment Scale (ESAS) was used to calculate the severity of pain, tiredness, drowsiness, nausea, appetite, shortness of breath, depression, anxiety, and best well-being. This is a two-page assessment tool that relies on patients to self-rate symptoms on a scale from 0 to 10, where 0 is no symptoms, and 10 is the worst possible presentation of the symptom. There is an option to report and rate one other symptom. On page two, there are drawings of an anterior and posterior body model with instruction to circle where the patient is experiencing pain.

In this study, seven out of nine symptoms were significantly improved with acupuncture; the exceptions were drowsiness and appetite. Acupuncture was found to be effective for the reduction and relief of symptoms that commonly affect patient quality of life (QOL). This is a good generalized study, but we need to get even more specific.

In 2008, an article from the *American Journal of Hospice and Palliative Medicine* (Standish, Kozak, and Cogdon 2008) declared that acupuncture is underutilized in hospice and palliative medicine. The conclusion was based on a literature search to identify clinical trials involving acupuncture, palliative care, hospice, chronic obstructive pulmonary disease, bone marrow, and cancer. Twenty-seven randomized controlled clinical trials of acupuncture were found, reporting on and including dyspnea, nausea and vomiting, pain, and xerostomia. Twenty-three of the 27 trials reported statistically significant results favoring acupuncture use for the conditions investigated. Acupuncture was found to be safe and clinically cost effective for management of common symptoms in palliative care and hospice patients.

If you repeated this search today, you would find additional volumes of reports that have reached the same conclusion. Despite the evidence, acupuncture is still underutilized in hospice and palliative care acupuncture.

One way that acupuncture professionals can help move hospice acupuncture forward as a specialty is to adopt the standardized Hospice Acupuncture Protocol form included in the Appendix of this book. There are also directions on how to send your results (minus any Health Insurance Portability and Accountability Act identifiers) to the National Association of Hospice and Palliative Care Acupuncturists.[2]

---

2   https://www.nahpca.com/research

Chapter 6

Assessment, Diagnosis, and Treatment of the Patients at the End of Life

In order to better serve patients at the end of life, practitioners of Asian Medicine must understand the complexity of symptoms that are part of the dying process. This chapter discusses problems unique to the treatment of hospice patients. Classic methods of diagnosis are not always reliable in patients with life-limiting illnesses. Practitioners who have not treated dying patients cannot make generalizations and must make assessments on a case-by-case basis and reassess before each treatment.

An emotional perspective on grief

Elisabeth Kübler-Ross wrote *Death and Dying* in 1969. The book described five stages of grief: denial, anger, bargaining, depression, and acceptance. The stages, now known as the Kübler-Ross model, outline a process for dealing with grief and tragedy for people who are suffering from terminal illness or catastrophic loss. Kübler-Ross is credited with bringing awareness to the mainstream for the need for greater sensitivity toward people with fatal disease. *Time* magazine said of the book, "It has brought death out of the darkness" (Hospice of Michigan 2009).

You will note that these stages relate directly to the five phases/ elements in Asian Medicine. This information can help you with your treatment plan and point selection. It can be used as an educational tool to teach the team members about the emotional healing properties of Asian Medicine. Most interdisciplinary team members have been introduced to the stages of grief as part of their training.

- *Denial* is the first stage and is usually temporary. The person is in a state of bewilderment, despite physical evidence or confirmation of a life-limiting illness.

- *Anger* generally follows denial. Typical feelings include envy and resentment toward healthy, energetic people. The ill person often states that life is not fair. During this stage, the patient is often full of rage and is difficult to care for.

- *Bargaining* is generally about the patient's hope for postponing or delaying death. The bargain may include changing habits, asking for more time, or promising to become more religious/spiritual. The patient may bargain with a higher power for some form of divine intervention.

- *Depression* is the stage in which the certainty of death begins to be comprehended. The patient grieves, often crying and becoming more withdrawn. They may become silent or refuse visitors—it is normal for them to disconnect from things representing love and affection.

- *Acceptance* means the patient begins to prepare for dying. They may state they are at peace and acknowledge that death is approaching. Some patients will want to be left alone or will have only small reserves of energy for communication with others. Due to physical and hormonal changes, feelings and physical pain may be non-existent. The dying struggle is over.

Elisabeth Kübler-Ross originally applied these stages to patients suffering from life-limiting illnesses. She later generalized the stages to any form of catastrophic personal loss. The stages can be, but are not always, sequential. People can switch between two or more stages, returning to one or more several times before moving on (Pajka 2007).

The grieving process is highly personal and often influenced by physiological changes. Some psychologists think that patients who fight harder against death are more likely to stay in denial. If a patient waits to confront death, it is seen by other psychologists as an adaptive behavior. The results of one study (Stanrock 2007) showed that patients who understood their purpose or special meaning faced less fear and despair in their last weeks of life than those who had not. Patients who considered themselves spiritual dealt with the depression stage more successfully than those who did not.

In Tibetan Medicine, a 2800-year-old tradition, you must pay attention to harmful influences such as hatred, ignorance, and jealousy that are connected in the mind and body. These influences are often expressed as lifelong issues that a patient may seek to resolve during the last months of their life. In the West, we are just beginning to understand how closely the mind and body are connected.

Again, because the focus of our treatment is to provide comfort, the point of this chapter is not for the practitioner to diagnose with a cure in mind. Instead, it is to help you to be more attuned to the changes you might observe in the normal course of your examination of patients near the end of life. Patients are dealing with fear of physical or emotional pain, fear of loneliness and abandonment, or an even greater fear that their life has been meaningless. Most importantly, your focus should be to assist them by releasing emotional blocks that would keep them from experiencing a peaceful death.

Note: The following is written in an instructive voice. It is meant to serve as a reminder of possible disease manifestations. There are many variations that diagnosis will reveal. In some patients, these signs may be subtle; in others, the change may be dramatic. The object here is not to interpret these changes, but simply to list common changes that occur in the patient who is approaching death.

Diagnosis by looking

Spirit: Is the patient thriving? *The Simple Questions* (a classic Chinese medical book) (Unschuld 1998) states this clearly: "If there is spirit the person thrives, if there is no spirit the person dies." If the mind is unclear, note the complexion, eyes, and state of breathing (see sections below for specific changes). Spirit is a yin characteristic. It is important to remember the phenomenon of false shen. When a patient has been minimally responsive and then suddenly awakens, maybe even opens their eyes, and begins talking, this is often false shen. The patient is using up the last reserves of the spirit. They often die within 48 hours of such activity.

Body: Note changes—are they happening over time or rapidly? Does the body seem to be suffering from cachexia (weight loss, wasting or atrophy of muscles, weakness or fatigue, and loss of appetite)? Do they have muscle stiffness or limited range of motion, weakness in limbs, loose skin, brittle bones, restlessness, muscle tension, shaking/jerking (often due to large amounts of opioids), or sweating? Can the patient maintain normal posture or alignment?

Demeanor: How does the patient move both the body and body parts? Are they experiencing dizziness or do they appear off-balance? Dying patients are usually less connected with physical surroundings and belongings and have diminished need or desire to communicate, and they may refuse to open their eyes. Patients may experience general restlessness—this is a sign that the oxygen supply to the brain is decreasing and the cerebral metabolism is slowing down. They may experience tremors, convulsions, fidgeting, pulling at bed linens, trying to get out of bed or a chair, or appear to be reaching for things that are not there. If the patient is anxious, they may have a pattern of symptoms including difficulty catching breath, sleeplessness, inability to relax, confusion, sweating, and difficulty paying attention or concentrating. It is important not to restrain the patient, but to limit physical contact and assess for spiritual distress. Often, distress can be diminished by playing calming music, or limiting outside noises and the number of people allowed at the bedside.

Head and face: Sagging of jaw occurs as a result of loss of facial tone. The overall facial complexion looks unhealthy. The color of the face may appear green, yellow, white, or black. Is it clear and shining, or is it dull (lifeless looking) or dry? It can change from appearing pale to dark or gray. Is there a specific area that is affected? This may correspond to disease in the major organ(s). The hair will appear dull as the skin dehydrates and vital oils are diminished. The patient may experience significant hair loss or premature graying.

Eyes: Does the shen shine through the patient's eyes? Note if the eyes move uncontrollably, with no inner vitality. Do the eyes look as if they are sinking? Are they glazed, dull, clouded, or do not appear clear? This often happens as the body loses moisture and the muscles weaken. Check for changes in the sclera—red spiral-shaped spots or other red, green, purple, blue, gray, or black spots may appear in the sclera. The whole sclera may turn red if there is internal bleeding, or yellow as the liver slows or ceases to function. Patients may become increasingly sensitive to light and ask to have lights dimmed or turned off, or they may cover their heads, or refuse to open their eyes. As muscle function weakens, the eyelids may stay partially or fully open, making the eyes very susceptible to dehydration. They often have a decreased or absent blink reflex.

Nose: Look for changes of color at the tip of the nose. The tip may appear dry and black if fire has taken over the stomach or large intestines. Cyanosis due to lack of oxygen will make the lips and nose appear blue, but a blue-green tip may be an indication of abdominal pain. If the patient has had prolonged anemia, the blood deficiency will make the tip appear white. Yellow on the tip appears in jaundiced patients as a manifestation of damp heat due to liver malfunction. If the patient has heart disease, the tip may appear red. Kidney and water impairment may make the tip of the nose appear gray.

Does the skin appear to be drooping? Again, this is an indication of loss of muscle tone. Does the patient have flaring at the nostrils? What about secretions? Do they have brittle, bloody, or dry crust inside or outside the nares? This may force them to breathe through the mouth. Another common change in patients is an increased sensitivity to odors, especially in patients who have had chemotherapy.

Ears: Hearing is the last sense to stop functioning. The patient may become overly sensitive to external stimulation and need quiet or only low-playing restful music. Look for variations in the ear lobes. Are they dry, withered, thin, or black? This may be a sign of kidney failure. Do they have swelling or pain due to internalized heat?

Mouth: Is the patient breathing only through the mouth? This may be an attempt by the body to get more oxygen. Their oral mucosa may become dry, dull, pale, or encrusted with secretions, or the skin may peel. Often, hospice patients are put on supplemental oxygen, which can exacerbate these problems. Humidity is usually added to increase patient comfort.

What is the color on and around their lips? Blue (cyanosis) is a sign of impending death. Note the skin on the lips—it may be cracked, cut, or dry and peeling. Are they coughing up mucus or blood? Does the tongue move freely or are they having difficulty speaking? Is there any drooling? Secretions often increase when the patient is actively dying.

Teeth and gums: Gums shrink due to patient dehydration and weight loss. As gums recede, there is more space between the teeth. The teeth may appear dry, become loose, and/or fall out. Dentures are too big for shrunken tissues, and can irritate or rub sores on gums. Changes in gums and teeth may cause redness, swelling, or bleeding. If a patient is anemic, the gums will appear pale.

Tongue: If the patient can stick out their tongue, you may wish to attempt a tongue diagnosis. It is important here to know that the internal changes that happen with dying patients are often so rapid, the tongue does not have time to register them, and traditional diagnostic techniques will not be accurate. Note variations in the tongue body shape and color, and in the coating and moisture level. Is the tongue cracked, quivering, or deviated? Most dying patients will have a dry tongue coated with yellow or sometimes black fur. It may also turn black after prolonged antibiotic treatments.

Throat: Patients may suffer from a red, sore, dry, or swollen throat due to oxygen use, decreased fluid intake, mouth breathing, and thrush or candidiasis. As muscles grow weaker and peristalsis diminishes, they may have difficulty swallowing. Secretions may collect in the back of the throat, making the patient choke. Oral suctioning may be used as a comfort measure to clear secretions, as patients often lose their gag reflex with their ability to swallow.

Limbs: Observe limbs for muscle wasting, tremors, possible sores, and skin tears. You may see discoloration or inflammation of joints (look for cyanosis on knees), contractures, or muscle spasm. Capillary refill in the nail beds becomes slower, often taking more than five seconds to refill.

Skin: In the end-of-life stage, the skin may appear dry and loose. If circulation and kidney function are diminished, the skin may look tight and shiny due to edema. Skin on joints can look dry and lacks luster. Some medications may cause patients to itch until they leave dry, white patches or red scratch marks. Skin over the larger joints (knees, elbows, ankles) may look blotchy. Mottled skin may be present on the hands, feet, legs, or arms. Elderly patients may have purple and blue raised venules (small veins) that appear behind their knees. As circulation decreases, skin may turn pale or appear blue as oxygenation slows. Yellow jaundiced skin reveals a failing liver. Skin appears wax-like when very near death.

There may be discoloration over the sacrum (like black magic marker spots) that becomes a large bedsore overnight. This is a Kennedy Terminal ulcer; it presents as pear-shaped and is colored red, yellow, or black. It is a sign of active dying, primarily seen in geriatric patients. Research shows most patients die in an 8–24-hour period after it appears.

Channels: Patients may have small, distended purple venules in areas specific to the channels (particularly the Blood Connecting Channels—one of the three types of very minute branches of the Connecting Channels, these areas are important to observe for visual diagnostic clues). Objective signs include purple spots, redness, white streaks, or skin rashes following a definite channel pathway. Flaccidity of the muscles, rigidity or hardness of the muscles, and cold or heat are also considered objective signs when found along the channels.

Diagnosis by hearing and smelling

Voice: Listen for changes in the voice quality; it may become weak or frail. The patient may stop talking or talk to people who are not there. The quality of speech may change from coherent to babbling, word salad (a mixture of random words), or sing-song.

Breathing: The patient may have restrictions or limitations on inhalation or expiration/exhalation due to muscle weakness, pain, tumors, diminished lung capacity, or fluid build-up. Dyspnea is exacerbated by these underlying disease processes. In general, respirations may increase if the patient's anxiety level rises due to these changes or emotional issues (such as fear of suffocation). The patient may snore loudly, or breathe in a barely audible manner when sleeping. Cheyne-Stokes breathing patterns are often a clinical sign of impending death. In this pattern, periods of apnea are alternated with periods of rapid breathing. Some patients will suffer from massive pleural effusions that may even cause the collapse of a lung.

Near the end of life, the patient often loses the ability to clear secretions, or lacks the strength to cough. Audible pattern changes in "the death rattle" include grunting, gurgling, or noisy congested breathing. Is the patient's breathing stertorous? In many cases, breathing gradually slows to terminal gasps sometimes known as "guppy breathing." It may sound as if the patient is working hard to breathe—a moaning sound may be heard with each breath.

Cough: As patients breathe through their mouths, they often develop a cough. Listen for coughing or weakened attempts to cough. The inability to cough or clear secretions will result in the grunting, gurgling, or noisy congested breathing mentioned above.

Auscultation (listening with a stethoscope) over the lung fields may reveal wheezes, stridor, rhonchi, rales, crackles, or crepitation.

Body smells: General body odors are related to the solid organs. A burned or burning smell is related to the heart. Sweet or fragrant smelling body odor signals the spleen's involvement in the disease process. Lungs produce a rank smell. Putrid or rotten smells are due to kidney disease. The liver is associated with a rancid or goatish odor. Breath, urine, and stools may also go through significant odor variations.

Bad breath: Due to changes in the lungs and breathing patterns, the breath takes on a metallic smell. Bad breath can be caused from sinus infections or from stomach heat. An absence of breath odor is due to internalized cold.

Stools: Constipation is frequently experienced by patients who have been on any form of pain medication. The stools may be dry and compressed and have little or no odor. The patient may moan or strain while attempting a bowel movement. Hardened stool can cause bleeding or impaction. Patients often have a serious decrease in appetite or they stop eating all together, making little to no stool. Bowel movements may slow or stop. An accumulation of gas may cause bowel sounds to increase temporarily or belching to occur.

Urine: Urinary frequency and burning occurs in some patients with bladder infections (common if the patient has been catheterized). Incontinence is common as patients lose muscle tone. If the patient gradually decreases all intake of fluids, urine output also decreases, becoming more concentrated, and has an ammonia smell. The patient may be unable to urinate. If this happens suddenly, it may be due to acute renal failure.

Diagnosis by asking

Some patients experience mental changes as they enter later stages of a disease process. They may not be reliable historians. Furthermore, speech patterns may become impaired, or there may be patients who simply cannot communicate verbally. Family members or other caregivers may have a more accurate picture of what is going on. Questions regarding the following symptoms may be added or omitted as relevant.

Chills and fever: The body loses its ability to control its temperature, and the patient may be hot one minute and cold the next.

Sweating: Note the location of perspiration, time of day, condition of illness, and quality of sweat. Body sweats may increase as the patient's heart rhythms change.

Head and body: Ask if the patient is experiencing headaches and dizziness. Is the patient experiencing disorientation, dreams of travel, visions or dreams of people who have already died, confusion about time, place, people, or family, or blurring of vision? These can occur as oxygen levels fluctuate in the brain. Remember, dyspnea is a subjective symptom, and even if the patient's SpO2[1] monitor is reading 100 percent, the patient may still report feeling short of breath and light-headed.

Thorax and abdomen: Common changes include increased heart rate, irregular rhythm, nausea and vomiting, and distension due to accumulation of gas. Ask and note the location (in respect to pathways of channels) of any pain.

Food and taste: Generally, the patient's appetite decreases. Some patients lose interest in eating and ask to be placed on an NPO status (nothing by mouth). Some simply refuse to eat, or want only sips or drops. Other patients may lose the ability to swallow, or may have to have thickened liquids in order to swallow. In these cases,

---

1   SpO2 is a medical abbreviation for peripheral oxygen saturation. This is measured by a small monitor that may be clamped to a finger or toe, or taped to an ear. The amount of oxygenated hemoglobin compared with all hemoglobin in the blood is displayed as a percentage on the device. It is meant to show arterial oxygenation at the end of the extremities. If this circulating hemoglobin is too low, that patient is often in need of supplemental oxygen.

patients are only given liquids on a swab to ease painful breakdown of oral tissues.

Stools and urine: Enquire about changes in size, frequency, or amount of stools. Has there been pus, mucus, blood, oozing, diarrhea, bloating or distension, cramping, nausea, or tenderness? If the patient is not eating, bowel movements normally cease within 48 hours of the last meal. Loss of control of bowel and bladder may occur days before, immediately prior to, or after the time of death, and is usually related to loss of sphincter control.

Sleep: The need for sleep often increases. Does the patient fatigue more easily and need naps? It is normal for patients to have dreams and visions of other people who have gone before them, and some have dreams of traveling. Sleeplessness or fear of sleep can be a sign of increasing anxiety. This is often treated with medications that cause further drowsiness.

Deafness and tinnitus: Has the patient's hearing become sensitive or impaired? Patients often hear things or voices that others are not hearing.

Thirst and drink: As patients near death, they may stop experiencing a sensation of thirst. Often, the family tries to make the patient drink when he or she has no desire. It is important for them to understand that forcing the patient to drink can lead to aspiration pneumonia, and they should not do it.

Pain: The patient with muscle and fat loss will have decreased absorption of drugs administered intramuscularly or subcutaneously. They could need a higher dose of pain medication if these routes are being used. Generally, as the patient nears death, pain decreases or ceases. Patients may stop needing pain medications.

Channels: Patients may report the following subjective symptoms along a channel: numbness, tingling, cold, heat, distension, pain, soreness, or dullness.

Gynecological conditions: Ask females who are still menstruating about any changes in frequency or duration of their cycles. Are they having an increase in pain or premenstrual symptoms? Variations on the amount, color, or quality of blood must be taken into account when considering the state of the patient's qi and blood. Any woman may have vaginal discharge issues as the body's pH changes.

Children's problems: In most cases, the parents or guardians of the child will be the ones answering the history questions. Remember, young children often do not have a concept of death. Acupuncture will not be used on most children due to fear of needles. Alternative treatments could include acupressure, seed, magnets, or a Manaka wooden hammer if the patient can tolerate it.

Diagnosis by feeling

It is important to remember to respect the wishes of patients. Often, at the end of life, patients withdraw or dislike being touched. It is best to complete the tactile part of the physical examination last, and limit palpation based on the patient's tolerance.

Skin: Palpable changes in the patient's skin can include areas that are hot or cold, loose or tight, and damp or dry. The skin may be tenting, pitting, sweating, or have inflammation over the joints. Elderly patients are susceptible to skin tears, and bedbound patients are at high risk for decubitus ulcers (bedsores). The patient may have a decreased sensation of touch.

Limbs: The dying patient's external temperature cools, and skin dries (particularly in patients with circulatory complications). In patients who have had a stroke, one side may be affected by such things as numbness and weakness.

Hands: As circulation decreases, the nails become dry and brittle and the hands feel cool or cold. The patient may have a lessening or loss of grip strength or dexterity.

Chest: Variations in heart beat can be felt over the chest wall of some patients. Retractions in the intercostal muscles may be felt and seen in patients who are struggling to breathe.

Abdomen: Bloating may occur or a patient may have a tumor that is easy to palpate. Hepatomegaly may be present so that the borders of the enlarged liver become easy to palpate. Several diseases can cause massive ascites.

Points: Sensations are generally dull when deficient, and sharp when excessive. Back Shu, Front Mu, Lower Sea, and Ashi points can be used for specific organ information—in general, patients will not appreciate point palpation when in end stage of life.

Pulse: As blood pressure decreases, pulses are more difficult to palpate; please see the section below for a complete discussion on pulses.

Pulse diagnosis

The following section is paraphrased from a translation of an ancient text (Unschuld 1998). Variations in pulse diagnosis for dying patients that were noted in the *Yellow Emperor's Classic of Internal Medicine* still hold true today.

In pulse diagnosis, the radial pulses can be felt on a portion of the lung meridian.

The pulses converge over an inch opening—lung points 7, 8, and 9. Lung 7 is the Luo connecting point of the lung. For simplicity, we will refer to pulse positions as noted in the *Nan Jing*:

	Cun (distal)		Guan (middle)		Chi (proximal)	
Left	Heart	Small Intestine	Liver	Gallbladder	Kidney	Urinary Bladder
Right	Lung	Large Intestine	Spleen	Stomach	Pericardium	Triple Warmer

The inch opening is on the distal, lateral wrist over the radius bone. It is a meeting point of the movement of all the organs through the pulses. The influences of the stomach are considered the basis for life. When food is supplied to the stomach, it is transmitted to the lungs, which supply the internal organs with influences. All the influences arrive at the one inch opening of the lung meridian and reflect their effects on the internal organs. If the influences sent out by the stomach are lost, the patient will die. That is a general rule.

These are the considerations in pulse diagnosis:

Does the movement of the pulses follow the course of heaven? Since the influences of man are the same as the course of heaven, if the movement in the vessels is contrary to the course of heaven then it does not reflect the influences of heaven. For instance, since summer is associated with Fire, the pulse should be surging during that season. A weak, thready pulse in summer would therefore be contrary to the course of heaven.

Successful healers of ancient times examined the influences emitted by the viscera in terms of the relationships of mutual generation and destruction among the phases. For instance, in case of an illness in the spleen, they feared a stringy movement in the vessels because Wood overcomes soil (Earth); and in case of an illness in the lung, they feared a surging pulse because Fire overcomes Metal.

Differentiate between pulse changes which fit the illness of the patient, and others that do not. If one has lost blood, the pulses should be calm and fine. If, in contrast, it is surging and large, this indicates that blood and other influences have been lost to the outside.

Pulse diagnosis cannot always correctly predict what kind of an illness someone has. It is also not always possible to know beforehand whether a person will die or survive, because the variations of the pulses are not regular.

Finally, the designations of illnesses are innumerable, yet they are reflected in merely a few dozen variations of the pulses. In the course of one single illness, those few dozen variations can all appear.

Even shortly prior to death, the pulse does not reflect true changes in organ functions because it takes a while for them to appear. One cannot safely determine when that person will die, except if the pulses in all six positions are fine and rapid for an extended period of time, then the patient will die. Also, the kidneys are for man what roots are for a tree, sources of continuous nourishment. If no movement associated with the kidneys can be felt in the vessels, the patient will soon die.

It is essential to utilize the other diagnostic methods: looking for changes in the patient's complexion, listening to the patient's voice and smelling her or his odors, and asking preferences for specific food flavors. If a patient cannot swallow food but vomits instead, the pulses can be similar to those of a healthy person for a while. If this goes on for a long time, the stomach will not receive nourishment and the pulses will undergo a violent change that no one will survive.

In general, though, if one investigates only the pulses or only the pathoconditions, any prediction concerning the successful or unfavorable outcome of an illness will be unreliable. The outcome of an illness can be determined only if both the pulses and the pathoconditions are taken into account. To make a correct prognosis, one must know which pathoconditions must not occur together with which pulses, and which pulses must not occur with which pathoconditions.

Pathoconditions are manifestations of an illness. If the illness is heat, the pathocondition is heat; if the illness is cold, the pathocondition is cold. That is a definite principle. There is an exception that all practitioners should know—pathoconditions and illnesses may contradict each other. For example, a patient is affected by cold, but on examination, his body is hot and has an aversion to heat. Being ignorant of this fact can lead to a mistake in the patient's treatment. If a practitioner prescribes drugs by only following the pathoconditions, the practitioner may end up giving a drug that hastens the patient's death.

In some disease processes, the change in pulses will not happen until the later stages of the illness. Also, the internal and external nature of an illness can differ, leading to a false reflection on the exterior. Comorbidities can lead to a confused picture of the pathoconditions as well. There are numerous other scenarios that may change the pulses and allow for incorrect interpretations.

In general, the practitioner needs to conduct a thorough examination and have a strong understanding of pathoconditions and pulse patterns in order to discern what is real. A partial or incomplete differentiation will lead to incorrect treatments or medications.

Another view from the Golden Mirror

That was not the only classic to deal with the pulses. The following translation is found in Bob Flaws's book *The Secret of Chinese Pulse Diagnosis* (1995). It is the second chapter of the "Rhymed Formula of the Essential Heart Methods of the Four Examinations" from the 34th juan of the *Yi Zong Jin Jian* (Golden Mirror of Ancestral Medicine).

Normal pulses and disease pulses
Have already been described in detail
Next will be handled [those dealing with] the expiry of the body
With the same sort of measure and weight [i.e. detail]

The pulse of the heart expiry
Is like the grasping of the hook on a belt.
[If it appears] agitated and racing like a spinning bean,
In one day one can die.

The pulse of the liver expiry
Is like touching the blade of a knife.
[If it appears] wiry like a newly strung bow,
Death will be in eight days.

The spleen expiry [pulse] is like a sparrow pecking.
It may also be like a roof leaking.

In addition, it may be like pouring water from a cup.
No rescue on the fourth day.

What is the dimension [of the pulse] of lung expiry?
It is like wind blowing through the hair
Or a feather striking the skin.
Three days and wailing.

What is [the pulse] of kidney expiry?
It is emitted like a taut cord
Or like tapping one's finger on a stone.
In four days it will happen.

The life [gate pulse] when it expires
Is like a fish hovering or shrimp swimming.
It may also arrive like a bubbling spring.
Nothing can persuade [the patient] to stay.

Chapter 7

Five Elements

In researching an appropriate generalized treatment model for hospice patients, one article by Ron Puhky, MD (2001), stood out. In his article, "Five Element acupuncture for terminal patients: A powerful intervention for dying well," he advocates for treatment of dying and grieving individuals with Five Element acupuncture, which is known to have a profound effect on emotions.

My initial introduction to the Five Elements began with education in Traditional Chinese Medicine. Over many years of practice and study, I experienced the benefits of both TCM and Five Element treatments for myself and for patients. This section of the book combines the major points of Dr. Puhky's article with clinical knowledge of Traditional Chinese Medicine, Western medicine, and hospice patient bedside care to offer the best information for treatment options.

The first written reference to the Five Elements or Five Phases can be found in the *Su Wen*, the first book of the *Huangdi Neijing* (*The Yellow Emperor's Inner Canon*, also known as *The Yellow Emperor's Classic of Internal Medicine*). In the Basic (or Simple) Questions, Huangdi discusses the use of Five Elements diagnosis in Asian Medicine. The practitioner must determine the elemental essence of the patient. Once this knowledge is gained, it is clear why the patient's illness is presenting in a particular pattern of disharmony. The focus is then on treating the causative or root factor of their illness, thereby restoring their elemental constitution to a balanced state.

Contrary to classic Five Element theory, in hospice patients this focus on the causative factor (CF) is not the key to treatments.

The dying patient's emotional and physical needs are considered first. Point selection is based on strengthening the element the patient needs to draw on the most to resolve their end-of-life issues and die at peace.

The sequences of the Five Elements are shown in Figure 7.1.

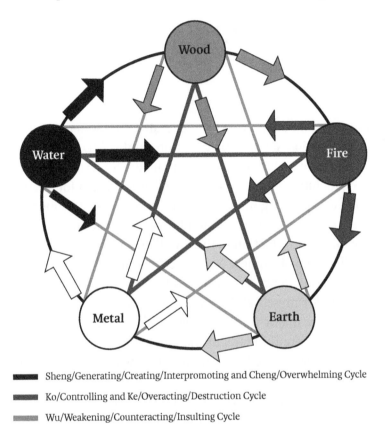

▬▬▬ Sheng/Generating/Creating/Interpromoting and Cheng/Overwhelming Cycle

▬▬▬ Ko/Controlling and Ke/Overacting/Destruction Cycle

▬▬▬ Wu/Weakening/Counteracting/Insulting Cycle

*Figure 7.1: The Interpromoting (Generating), Interacting (Controlling),
and Counteracting (Insulting) sequences of the Wuxing/Five Elements*

The following is a review of the Five Element conflicts and resolutions regarding emotional issues surrounding dying.

Water: *Fear and survival issues*

Fear of death and the unknown. Fear paralyzes and blocks healing and adaptive energies. Fear increases physical and psychological pain.

Strengthening Water gives patients the courage of the warrior, the hero, so they can face and deal with incredible odds. Water points can be used to tap into big reservoirs of spirit—the storehouse of ancestral energies and wisdom, and inner knowing.

Physiologically and energetically, it is connected to the natural processes of letting go and dying with more ease and less pain.

Wood: *Anger and injustice people feel when facing death*

Treatments release anger and open the pathway to forgiveness of the self and others. This allows a feeling of completion and closure that creates a sense of peace which enables the patient to effectively plan and carry out their dying process.

Metal: *Denial, not accepting, and refusal to let go of life*

Treatment helps the patient to soften and relax, feeling and acknowledging the richness and worth of life. This allows them to accept the inevitability of dying and to be present through farewells, tears, grief, and loss. The end result is letting go with greater ease, and dying with grace and fewer regrets.

Many patients die in the early morning hours between 3am and 7am, which is the time of Metal. Through the lungs, Metal allows the patient to grasp their deeper spiritual essence. Breathing, the patient connects outwardly to heaven and inwardly to their spiritual essence. The last breath completes the soul's movement back to pure, formless spirit.

Earth: *Obsession, self-absorption, worry, anxiety, and feeling of victimization*

Resolving Earth energies gives the patient a sense of place, home, and comfort within our human community. The element Earth represents not only where we belong, but to whom we belong— our family, our friends, our tribe. When balanced, this element allows us to embrace our internalized mother and to experience the universal principle of the Earth as our Mother. At peace with creation, patients can express satisfaction with the works they have created and gratitude for all of their blessings. As worry dissolves, the patient becomes grounded and centered in the flow of life. Accepting the continuity of life's process leads to a sense of completion that allows for a peaceful death.

Fire: *Despair, loneliness, isolation, contracted spirit, and feeling unlovable*

In balance, Fire allows us to feel love, joy, and freedom to expand our consciousness into our spiritual center, which connects us to the unity of all life. The heart holds our shen, our deathless unchanging nature—our immortal essence. As death nears, a person moves into Fire. By resolving Fire imbalances, a person can move naturally and joyfully into the next stage of their journey, connecting with their dearly departed, teachers, saints, sages, immortal ancestors, and their sense of the divine and the whole cosmos. Often, after a near-death experience, patients express a sense of relief and readiness in feeling embraced by those who have gone before. Opening to heart energy, patients can express their true love of family and friends and say their goodbyes. This heartfelt expression allows the patient to rest in their shen, experiencing a sense of completion and appreciation for the joy of the world as they depart from it.

Principles of treatment

The pulses may not be good indicators of the overall internal state of an individual. Initially, pulse diagnosis may be able to give specific information about the state of each element; later they may give feedback on how point choices and treatments are working.

Treatments must be adjusted based on the patient's emotional state, elemental needs, and pulse analysis. In cases of extreme agitation, sedation can be attempted using the Four Gates—LI 4 (Hegu) and Liv 3 (Taichong), with Du/GV 20 (Baihui). It is important to remember it may be impractical or even dangerous to use needles. Electroacupuncture pens/pointers, ear probes, magnets, and dull-tipped massage tools, as well as acupressure, are all acceptable alternatives to needles.

Pulses that are chaotic as the patient nears death (as discussed in the pulse diagnosis section) should be treated with spirit points. The intense and unorganized quality of the pulse can be diminished and balanced by using the spirit points. Husband/Wife imbalances (where the right-hand pulses are stronger and more aggressive than the left) are indirectly treated with spirit points to equalize their strengths and promote a healthy state.

Treatments should end with distal command points leaving pulses calmed and balanced. Clinical signs may be subtle. The patient may communicate results directly by mentioning a decrease in pain and anxiety, or indirect feedback may be expressed by relaxed breathing, or a decrease in restless movement, or a caregiver's observations.

Patients may require acupuncture treatments either daily or every two to three days when beginning. It is important to educate the patient and their close friends or family on how to determine when further treatments may be needed. The friends and family need to communicate the patient's degree of pain or anxiety, confusion or restlessness, and the quality of her or his interactions with loved ones.

When the dying person reaches a certain point of equilibrium and is in communication with their spirit, they can tap into the natural process of dying. If their heart is open, humor and joking with loved ones, or other expressions of happiness, can lead to deeper, heartfelt final communications. This process has its own flow, purpose, meaning, and solace.

In review, acupuncture is a specific and effective way to aid the dying process. When our qi is balanced, we have an innate, natural process for connecting with our spirit, expanding our capacity for healing and "letting go" of the body. Acupuncture helps to improve the patient's inner experience while diminishing their physical distress. Acupuncture treatments are powerful medicine in hospice care. Their use has already led to the development of new insights and understandings about the dying process.

Treatment techniques

In palliative care acupuncture, the primary needle technique is gentle reinforcing or tonification. Insert the needle with a slight angle toward the direction of energetic flow of the meridian. Advance slowly to the proper depth for de qi to be obtained. *It is important to remember that shallow insertion is advisable on face, head, or back points. Shallow insertion is also recommended on all points for individuals suffering from deficiency of qi and blood, or with weak constitutions—such as infants or the elderly.* Once qi is felt, rotate the needle clockwise 180°, then withdraw the needle rapidly after two or three seconds and seal the point with a cotton ball and finger pressure.

Reducing or sedation is used less often. Insertion is quick, with slight angulations against the direction of flow of the energy in the meridian. The needle is rotated 180° counterclockwise, then retained for 15–20 minutes. Withdraw the needle slowly with a shaking motion to enlarge the hole and let the pathogenic factor exit. Do not seal the point.

If you are using moxa, it should be direct or open non-scarring moxibustion. Most points are treated using three to five hand-rolled, pea-sized moxa cones. Apply one cone directly on the point to be treated and then replace it, when the patient first feels a burning discomfort. If you are working with patients in facilities, there may be restrictions about smoke or fire, as well as fire alarms that are triggered by smoke. Do not use moxa on patients who are on oxygen or who have breathing difficulties. Oxygen is combustible and must not be used around open flames. Moxa in liquid, gel, spray, or plaster form may be used as an alternative. *Remember, a patient's pain perception is often compromised and careful observation is required, so do not burn the skin!* Moxibustion can be followed with needle reinforcement as described above. Generally, it is best to treat spirit points first.

Hospice Acupuncture Protocol

The basic protocol for hospice treatments is to start with spirit points to bolster the patient's inner strength. The ancestor points are needled next to evoke peace by connecting the patient to their sense of the sacred. Follow that with points to dispel residual fears. The treatment can be finished with points for letting go. This protocol is dependent on the patient's condition. This is by no means a replacement for a full assessment and sound clinical judgment by the practitioner to custom fit the treatment to the patient. Alternative points may be used as the patient can tolerate or as the practitioner sees fit, as can alternative applications such as acupressure or moxibustion.

Spirit points

Start the treatment by applying direct moxibustion to one of the large general spirit points of the Kidney: K 23 (Shenfeng) (Spirit Seal), K 24 (Lingxu) (Spirit Burial Ground), or K 25 (Shencang) (Spirit Storehouse). Treating these big reservoirs of spirit will ease the patient's fear; stimulation on these points delivers a sense of calmness and inner strength.

Treat the heart and connect with your patient there by treating the shen. Needling the Front (Mu) point of the heart, Ren/CV 14 (Great Deficiency), is very potent at this time. UB 44 (39) (Shentang) (Spirit Hall), the transporting point of the heart, and H 1 (Jiquan) (Utmost Source) are useful for heart matters. H 7 (Shenmen) (Spirit Gate) opens the gate to the shen and can be used repeatedly to keep the gate open.

Ancestor points

When a patient is experiencing agitation or depletion which is reflected by their pulses, Du/GV 20 (Baihui) (One Hundred Meetings) should be reduced/sedated or reinforced/tonified respectively. This point and the extra points of Sishencong are all the assembly of the ancestor points, the place where the soul leaves the body. These points correspond to the location of the crown chakra, and treating them evokes peace, comfort, and stability of the mind and spirit. In this state, the patient can connect to departed loved ones and his or her holy or spiritual guides, angels, sages, and saints.

SI 11 (Tianzong) (Heavenly Ancestor) can be used in much the same manner, as it is linked to the shen as the heart's paired (yang) organ. The triple heater and especially SJ 7 (Huizong) (Assembly of Ancestors) has a major effect on calling up archetypal and ancestral energies.

Points for fear

Treating Water points, especially kidney points, eases fear. Reinforce/tonify K 21 (Youmen) (Dark Gate) to reduce residual fears after treating the above-mentioned spirit points. Follow by using Ren/CV 14 (Juque) (Great Palace)—the Front (Mu) point of the heart—if you have not previously used it. Next apply direct moxibustion over those two points. Later, K 20 (Tonggu) (Through the Valley) may be added; and source point K 3 (Taixi) (Greater Mountain Stream) can be used alone, or added to the above points for unresolved fear. Water points UB 57 (Chengshan) (Supporting Mountain) and UB 61 (Pucan) (Servant's Aide), and also the source point UB 64 (Jinggu) (Capital Bone), may be substituted for letting go of fear.

Points for letting go

Metal and Wood elements can be used when patients are clinging to life and have not yet accepted the idea of dying. Lung and Large Intestine points promote stillness and strengthen the will, aiding in the smooth evolution of the dying process. Source points in the yang organs, LI 4 (Hegu) (Joining of the Valleys) and GB 40 (Qiuxu) (Wilderness Mound), can be used to expel pathogenic factors when there is an Excess pattern. In the yin organs, Lu 9 (Taiyuan) (Very Great Abyss) and Liv 3 (Taichong) (Supreme Rushing) will reflect the state of Original Qi (look for changes on the skin over the point).

Other Metal points LI 17 (Tianding) (Heavenly Vessel), LI 18 (Futu) (Support and Rush Out), and Lu 3 (Tainfu) (Heavenly Palace) help the patient reconnect to spirit. Treating Wood points relaxes the need for control and promotes letting go of anger, struggle, and any sense of unfairness or injustice that is disturbing the individual.

GB 40 (Qiuxu) (Wilderness Mound) and Liv 13 (Zhangmen) (Gate of Brightness), or Liv 14 (Qimen) (Gate of Hope), can be used together with reduction/sedation to initiate change and give hope. Reinforcing/tonifying Liv 3 (Taichong) (Supreme Rushing) will bring the patient a sense of hope and strength.

Other points for consideration

Miriam Lee (1992) has written an excellent book recommending the following points as a treatment protocol: St 36 (Zusanli), LI 4 (Hegu), LI 11 (Quchi), Lu 7 (Lieque), and Sp 6 (Sanyinjiao). These points can be used for general relaxation and are excellent points to treat patients and their families. They lend themselves well to a community approach.

Treatment protocol samples

These samples are meant as examples only. They are not meant to be used to replace a thorough examination and clinical diagnosis of the patient. However, it is important to remember that the aim of hospice-based acupuncture is to encourage the patient's emotional release and support the resolution of issues that would prevent the patient from having a peaceful death.

The patient is expressing a deep sense of negativity and fear. Everything feels like a struggle.

- *Spirit point:* K 25 (Shencang) builds up the patient's spiritual reserve. Tonify.

- *Ancestor point:* Du/GV 20 (Baihui) clears the mind and lifts the spirit by helping the patient connect with the strength and wisdom of ancestors who have gone before. Tonify.

- *Point for fear:* Ren/CV 14 (Juque) reduces residual fear. Tonify, and then follow with direct moxa, if possible.

- *Point for letting go:* Liv 3 (Taichong) releases general nervous tension and gives the patient a sense of hope. Tonify.

The patient is expressing anger toward family members and states that he wants to be left alone.

- *Spirit point:* UB 47 (42) (Hunmen) is especially good for Wood CF, as it roots the ethereal soul and releases long-standing resentments. May be tonified or reduced as needed.

- *Ancestor point:* Shishencong descends rebellious qi and subdues anger. Reduce.

- *Point for fear:* K 20 (Tonggu) releases fear of facing death, being alone, and suicide. Anger often stems from fear of loss and resentment toward healthy people. Tonify.

- *Point for letting go:* Liv 13 (Zhangmen) gives the patient hope and allows them to move on and plan for the future. Reduce.

Table 5.1 is a review and summary of the Hospice Acupuncture Protocol, and may be used in clinical applications.

Table 5.1: Five Phases/Elements correspondences

Element	WOOD	FIRE	EARTH	METAL	WATER
Yin organ	Liver	Heart	Spleen	Lung	Kidney
Yang organ	Gallbladder	Small Intestine	Stomach	Large Intestine	Urinary Bladder
Sense organ	Eyes	Tongue	Mouth	Nose	Ears
Emotion	Anger	Joy/Shock	Worry	Sadness/Grief/Sorrow	Anxiety/Fear
Body tissue	Sinews	Blood Vessel	Muscles	Skin	Bone
Climate qi	Wind	Heat	Dampness	Dryness	Cold
Color	Green	Red	Yellow	White	Black
Season	Spring	Summer	Late Summer	Autumn	Winter
Sound	Shouting	Laughing	Singing	Crying	Groaning
Taste	Sour	Bitter	Sweet	Spicy	Salty
Issue	Sense of injustice, struggle, and incompletion of life	Despair, loneliness, isolation, feeling unlovable, and contracted spirit	Obsession, self-absorption, anxiety, and feeling of victimization	Loss, denial, excessive clinging, spiritual emptiness, and many regrets	Terror of death, and fear of non-existence
Elemental gift/ Therapeutic influence	Forgiveness of self and others, relaxation, and completion	Opens to love and relationships, joy, beauty, unity, god, and self-confidence	Comfort, sense of family, belonging, contentment, and gratitude for life	Accepting impermanence and death, letting go, reconciliation to spirit, and big mind	Courage, will, stillness, calm, and reassurance
Regular meridian points	Liv 3, Liv 13, Liv 14, GB 40	H 1, H 7, SI 11, P 3, P 4, P 6, P 7, SI 4, SI 7, SI 10	Sp 3, Sp 6, Sp 21, St 36, St 40, St 42	Lu 1, Lu 3, Lu 7, Lu 9, LI 4, LI 11, LI 17, LI 18	K 3, K 20, K 21, K 23, K 24, K 25, UB 44 (39), UB 47 (42), UB 52 (47), UB 57, UB 61, UB 64
Other points	Ren/CV 14				Du/GV 20, Sishencong

Chapter 8

Channel Points for Consideration

R eading acupuncture literature can expose you to a variety of synonyms that may cause confusion and frustration. To assist you with the terminology here, check the Glossary for Point Nomenclature at the end of the book. The following point functions are drawn from Brassington 1998; Macicocia 1989; Lianyue *et al.* 1987; and Shanghai College of Traditional Medicine 1981, as well as years of clinical experience.

Wood

Liver: Foot Jue Yin

Liv 3 (Taichong) (Great Pouring, Supreme Rushing, Bigger Rushing)

> Shu/Stream/Transporting point; Tu/Earth point; Yuan/Primary/ Source point

Taichong promotes the smooth flow of liver qi by subduing liver yang. This is a good point for expelling interior wind and promoting a profound sense of happiness and calmness. It allows patients to relax their need for control and helps them to release anger, impatience, struggle, and feelings that life is being unjust or unfair. It helps to soothe communication, resentment, and difficulties due to intolerance in relationships. Liv 3 (Taichong) may be used for agitation (best in combination with LI 4 (Hegu) and Du 20 (Baihui)), strong feelings of frustration, hypertension, irritability, and quick-tempered angry outbursts. It can treat stress, depression, mania, and generalized nervous tension. Liv 3 (Taichong) also calms spasms.

Liv 13 (Zhangmen) (System's Door, Chapter Gate, Camphorwood Gate, Gate of Brightness)

> Crossing/Coalescent/Point of Intersection with Gallbladder Channel; Hui/Gathering/Meeting/Influential point for the 5 Zang/Yin Organs; Mu/Front/Alarm/Collecting point of Spleen

This is an excellent gate point to initiate change when a patient has feelings of hopelessness, spiritlessness, and not being able to go on with life. It works on all levels—mind, body, and spirit. This powerful point helps the patient to have hope, vision, and a desire to plan for the future when used in combination with Liv 14 (Qimen). Because of its association with the spleen, it benefits both the spleen and stomach and relieves retention of food.

Liv 14 (Qimen) (Expectation's Door, Gate of Hope, Cyclic Gate)

> Crossing/Coalescent/Points of Intersection with the Spleen and Yin Wei/Linking Channel; Exit point; Mu/Front/Collecting point of the Liver

This point has many of the same effects as Liv 13 (Zhangmen) in that it releases anger, frustration, feelings of injustice, and the need to control. It is good for treating the patient who is totally blocked—no direction, no hope, no fulfillment, no joy in life or achievements, just mental torture and no desire to go on. Opening the Gate of Hope allows the patient to move on. This point cools the blood, promotes smooth flow of liver qi, and benefits the stomach. It can be used to treat mental disorders induced by high fevers. Treatment with this point and Liv 13 (Zhangmen) opens a new qi cycle allowing for flexibility and renewed hope for possibilities, plans, and life.

Gallbladder: Foot Shao Yang
GB 40 (Qiuxu) (Mounds of Ruins, Wilderness Mound, Hill Ruins)

Yuan/Primary/Source point

This point is also known as the Ancestor's Burial Mound—a place to connect to their knowledge and wisdom in a way that supports strength of character and clarity of decision making. This is a good point to use when a patient expresses uncertainty, indecision, or feeling muddled in thoughts. It gives the patient a feeling of mental strength and certainty, which promotes a feeling of calmness when vital judgments must be made. Much like the liver points above, this point can be used for relaxing the need for control. It also promotes the smooth flow of liver qi and clears gallbladder heat, which leads to letting go of anger, frustration, struggle, and feelings of injustice or unfairness. Physically, it treats headaches, sighing, and abdominal distension, and promotes faster healing after surgeries.

Fire
Heart: Hand Shao Yin
H 1 (Jiquan) (Summit's Spring, Utmost Source, Supreme Spring, Highest Spring)

Entry point

This point allows us to understand that we are all one and that outside energy is inside energy; there is no difference. It keeps the gate of shen open so that the emperor, god, or supreme controller within us can communicate to the God outside us. The supreme controller brings cohesion to all of the officials. This point is where we are connected to all life or energy as we are part of all energy or all that is living. If this connection is lost, a person will begin to exhibit signs of uncertainty or chaotic thoughts and may become hysterical or panic-stricken. H 1 clears empty heat. It nourishes heart yin to help resolve feelings of struggling to survive or a strong desire toward isolation, or of being unlovable or conversely unable to feel love or express compassion, warmth, and joy. Physically, Jiquan treats paralysis, numbness, mental restlessness, and insomnia.

H 7 (Shenmen) (Spirit's Door, Spirit Gate, Mind Door)

Son/Sedation/Reducing point; Shu/Stream/Transporting point; Yuan/Primary/Source point

Shenmen is a major body point and the most important heart point because it can be used in any heart pattern to calm the mind. This point allows a person to experience opposites without getting stuck by regulating the opening and closing of the gate of shen. By primarily nourishing the heart blood, it lends stability to someone who has "given up the ghost" (acting depressed or feeling hopeless). These patients will present as appearing dull, slow, lacking interest, being too tired to talk, and/or avoiding social situations. Conversely, it can treat heart blood deficiency to stabilize patients in exceedingly high spirits with anxiety, excessive worrying, and insomnia. It can treat patients who are feeling stressed, jumpy, tense, easily upset with palpitations and emotional hypertension, which can lead to being out of control and resulting in mental exhaustion, poor memory, shutting off, collapse, or mania. Chronic illness depletes the spirits, walling patients off from life—this is the best point for stressful situations. This point opens the orifices, reawakens the spirit, aids mental capacity, and strengthens the will. It is also used in palliative care to increase salivation.

Small Intestine: Hand Tai Yang
SI 11 (Tianzong) (Heaven's Ancestor, Heaven's Attribution, Celestial Gathering)

Ancestor point

This Ancestor point is good for promoting a slow, positive mental change. It is linked to shen as the heart's paired organ. The most powerful mental point on the Small Intestine meridian, it brings clarity of thoughts and peaceful tranquility when stimulated. This deep-reaching spiritual point enables the patient to connect with the wisdom of departed elders, ancestors, or other spiritual beings. By tapping into this support, the patient is able to sort (once chaotic) thoughts and make clear decisions. Physically, it can treat the shoulder, improving range of motion in painful obstructive syndrome and metaphysically extending the patient's reach.

Pericardium: Hand Jue Yin
P 3 (Quze) (Marsh on/at the Bend, Crooked Marsh)

He/Sea point; Shui/Water point

This point clears heat, cools blood, and expels heart-fire poison. Patients with heart-fire poison often report being easily frightened or having fear of meeting new people and/or of water. They sometimes dream of water or fire raging out of control, and often have whole body heat, thirst, and febrile conditions, with trembling or convulsions. This point moves and regulates blood by dispelling stasis; it pacifies the stomach to relieve pain and stop vomiting; and it opens the orifices. It is excellent for treating bipolar presentations, exhaustion, suicidal ideations, and overly sensitive patients. It calms the minds of patients suffering from extreme excitement, vexation, agitation, fright, or anxiety, which cause hypertension-related headaches, irritability, dizziness, or mania.

P 4 (Ximen) (Cleft Door, Cleft Gate, Gate of Qi Reserve, Gate of the Crevice)

Xi/Cleft/Accumulation point

Ximen is a very strong mental point that strengthens the mind, alleviates fears, and bolsters courage by treating heart deficiency. By regulating and cooling blood, it pacifies the heart to bring a sense of serenity and peace to calm the spirit. When blood is regulated, qi is regulated, the heart rhythm becomes regular; the heart is calm and acute conditions are relieved, so pain stops. Treating with this point removes obstructions from the channel, opens the chest, and allows the diaphragm to expand. It nourishes, fortifies, and stabilizes the spirit in people who feel they have no reserve left. This point raises spirit qi to make the patient smile again. As an alternative source point, it can be used for psychic imbalances to treat fear of people or strangers, depression, mania, breakdowns, and hysteria.

P 6 (Neiguan) (Inner Gate, Inner Pass, Inner Frontier Gate)

Luo/Connecting point with the San Jiao Channel; Xi/Confluent/ Opening/Meeting point of the Yin Wei/Linking Channel

This point regulates heart qi and blood and calms fire, thus decreasing palpitations and anxiety. It opens the chest to treat feelings of fullness and difficulty breathing. The Inner Gate calms the mind and is most useful for treating depression of the highest degree; it also treats insomnia by promoting sleep. It is a good point to stimulate when a patient is suffering from fatigue or grief, and withdrawing from life and relationships. It allows the patient a heartfelt journey inward, helping them to define what they want out of life. This point may be used to restore balance between the body and mind and give the patient hope of getting better.

Physically, Neiguan can be used to increase the patient's quality of life by regulating terminal yin, increasing coordination, and decreasing pain, leucopenia, dizziness, and weakness. It regulates and clears the triple burner and harmonizes the stomach. It is used in palliative care to decrease nausea (both frequency and severity), appetite suppression, and emesis episodes; this leads to a decreased need for antiemetic drugs and an increase in salivation.

P 7 (Daling) (Great Hill, Great Mound, Big Tomb)

Son/Sedation/Reducing point; Shu/Stream/Transporting point; Tu/Earth point; Yuan/Primary/Source point

Historically, this point was used as the source point of the heart to ground fire, clear heat, and calm the mind. It has a strong effect for women who are dealing with emotional problems such as sadness, fear, worry, or anxiety from troubled relationships or breakups. The Great Hill refers to the burial mound of the emperors. It calms the spirit and brings a sense of security by allowing the patient to tap into the nurturing source energy of their forbearers. By calling on this great reserve, the patient can see issues more clearly. This point clears the heart fire to treat mental problems such as mania, anxiety, and mental restlessness. Daling may be used for patients with weak nerves, instability of moods, palpitations, insomnia, irritability, forgetfulness, weeping, incessant laughter, panic attacks, or hysteria. It can also be used for gastritis as it harmonizes the stomach and expands the chest.

San Jiao: Hand Shao Yang
SJ 4 (Yangchi) (Yang Pond, Yang Pool)

Yuan/Primary/Source point

The Yang Pool relates to the water analogy of the San Jiao/Triple Warmer. Drawing from the Yang Pool benefits and tonifies original qi. It can be used to treat all chronic diseases causing deficiencies, including kidney deficiency. It raises the weakened patient's energy to alleviate tiredness and can re-establish warmth and harmony.

Yangchi dispels wind, disperses heat, relaxes sinews, and is especially good for occipital headaches. It tonifies, penetrating and directing vessels, promotes circulation, and reduces hypertension. This point removes obstructions and clears the channels, including painful obstruction of the arm and shoulder. It regulates the stomach and promotes fluid transformation and excretion.

SJ 7 (Huizong) (Meeting of the Clan, Assembly of Ancestors, Converging Channels, Convergence and Gathering)

Ancestor point; Xi/Cleft/Accumulation point

This assembly point of the ancestors, like all accumulating points, can be used in acute patterns. It clears heat and relieves stagnation. It soothes by removing obstruction, thus freeing up channel qi. In excess patterns, it is used to stop pain in the eyes, eyebrows, ears, and temples. Mentally, it is effective for giddiness and confused or chaotic thoughts. Spiritually, stimulation of this point calls up archetypal and ancestral energies and anchors the patient with feelings of support and stability. Drawing on supreme wisdom, and feeling back in control, the patient experiences a sense of tranquility and calm peace. It can be needled often without adverse effects.

SJ 10 (Tianjing) (Heaven's Well, Heavenly Well, Celestial Well)

He/Sea/Uniting point; Tu/Earth point; Son/Sedation/Reducing point

This point treats physical, spiritual, and emotional pain. It relaxes tendons, dispels stagnation, and unblocks channels to relieve painful obstruction. By dispelling wind and clearing heat, Tianjing stops pain and stiffness and treats migraines. By regulating nutritive and defensive qi and resolving dampness and phlegm, it treats digestive and lymphatic disorders to improve the patient's overall feeling of wellness. This point refers to an inexhaustible well of heavenly qi that can be tapped to calm and strengthen the spirit and stabilize the mind. This is a deep-reaching point that promotes clarity and beauty for the patient who has lost their sense of self or spiritual connection with their concept of God. Because this point can ground fire, it treats emotional problems such as insecurity, restlessness, and deep sorrow. It evokes a sense of serenity and peace by making people feel held and secure.

Earth

Spleen: Foot Tai Yin

Sp 3 (Taibai) (Supreme White, Greater White, Most White)

Shu/Stream/Transporting point; Tu/Earth point; Yuan/Primary/ Source point

Use this point when a patient is confused or having muddled thinking. This is an excellent point for promoting mental clarity by stimulating the brain and fortifying the memory. By strengthening the spleen and resolving dampness, this point alleviates mental exhaustion, including vague feelings of heaviness, dullness, and overall tiredness, a lack of ability to concentrate, blurred vision, and insomnia. It resolves dampness in all three burners to relieve feelings of fullness in the chest and chronic backache. It can also stabilize the bowels and treat difficult and cloudy urination.

Sp 6 (Sanyinjiao) (Three Yin Meeting, Three Yin Crossings)

Crossing/Coalescent/Points of Intersection with (Three Leg Yin) Kidney and Liver Channels

This is one of the most important acupuncture points. It nourishes blood to calm the mind and allay irritability. It can treat nervous tension, including fear, hypersensitivity, restlessness, and insomnia. It can be used for deep depression, for people feeling desperate, or as if they have met their limit, but it must be used with caution in volatile people. Sanyinjiao is a good point to stop pain by stimulating blood movement, eliminating stasis, cooling blood, and soothing liver qi. By moving qi, it alleviates tiredness. Sanyinjiao is a major point for treating abdominal pain, irregular stools, and gynecological problems.

Sp 21 (Dabao) (Big Wrapping, Great Enveloping, Great Embrace, Encircling Glory, General Control)

Luo/Connecting point of the Great Channel of the Spleen

Dabao moves blood (in the Blood Connecting Channels) to treat generalized pain, muscular pain, tiredness, or weakness. It may be used for patients living with general disorders, including feelings of being fractured or out of contact.

Stomach: Foot Yang Ming
St 36 (Zusanli) (Three Miles of the Foot, Three Measures on the Leg)

Earth point; Lower He/Sea point of Stomach (Sea of Food/Grains); He/Sea/Uniting point

This point is potent in fighting disease by preventing attacks from exterior pathogenic factors. It increases overall resistance to disease, and when used with moxibustion, it increases the patient's white blood count. It can be used with people suffering from chronic illness or debilitating diseases to regulate defensive qi and blood. It moves and revitalizes energy to strengthen the body and the mind. This point is a means for the patient to gain endurance to move on, mentally, physically, and spiritually. It is the main point to tonify post-heaven qi.

Zusanli is a point of the sea of nourishment or food, so it can be used for any eating disorder, including emaciation from general deficiency. It benefits the stomach, spleen, and intestines by regulating nutritive qi and expelling cold, wind, and dampness. It raises yang to brighten the eyes. Treating with this point can resolve edema and painful obstruction of the knee.

St 40 (Fenglong) (Abundance and Prosperity, Abundant Bulge, Bountiful Bulge)

Luo/Connecting with the Divergent Channel of the Spleen

St 40 is a reserve of abundant energy—it generally raises energy. Fenglong allows people to have a sense of the harvest from life's toil. It treats depression and helps with feelings of dissatisfaction. This point works on the mental side of Earth and calms the spirit for thought patterns, including ghosts, obsessions, or feeling ungrounded and not in contact with the earth. It can be used to eliminate phlegm that mists the mind, causing mental disturbances or simply dizziness and fuzziness of the brain. It calms the mind and can be used in cases including anxiety, fears, and phobias. It resolves dampness in the brain. Treating with St 40 helps with tightness of the epigastrium and "knots" or "butterflies" in the stomach. It relaxes and opens the chest and resolves lung dampness to soothe breathing and treat asthmatic symptoms. Research confirms that it is most often used in palliative care to decrease excessive sputum and breathlessness.

St 42 (Chongyang) (Rushing Yang, Pouring Yang)

Exit point; Yuan/Primary/Source point

This is an excellent point for promoting mental stability and calming the mind. It is most useful for maniac presentations of mental illness which may include loud, fast talking or singing, exaggerated behaviors, walking aimlessly without true focus, removing clothes, or simply being unable to maintain normal emotional control. This point removes obstruction from the channel, and may be used with SJ 4 to tonify the spleen and stomach. Needle Chongyang with *caution* to avoid puncturing blood vessels.

Metal
Lung: Hand Tai Yin
Lu 1 (Zhongfu) (Central Residence, Middle Palace, Central Treasury)

> Crossing/Coalescent/Point of Intersection with Spleen Channel; Entry point; Mu/Front/Collecting/Alarm point of the Lungs

Passing through the middle palace is how one arrives at the inner palace, where God resides. This point is about opening the spirit to bring a renewed sense of joy and inspiration to life. Use this point when a person is stuck or depressed and doesn't feel good about themselves or life; or when a patient cannot accept compliments or praise and belittles respect. This point gives inspiration—it allows patients to reconnect with the essence of life by getting them back in touch with the breath of heaven. It brings in the light of the heavens to allow the patient to experience the richness and joy of every breath. It can be combined with Ren/CV 17 (Danzhong) and Lu 7 (Lieque) to open the chest for cases of melancholy or depression.

This is a very good point for treating grief because it goes directly to the source of grief, releasing emotional blocks to help move the person through his or her tears. This point moves and regulates lung qi—treating stagnation and opening up the chest energy to allow the patient to experience the breath of heaven.

This point is in close proximity to the lungs, where qi is infused and converged. Zhongfu is best used in excess patterns for acute manifestations, not root problems. By opening up the chest energy, it can decrease breathlessness and treat coughing caused by retention of phlegm, excess sputum, asthma, pain in the chest, shoulder, and back, and fullness of the chest.

Lu 3 (Tianfu) (Heaven's Residence, Heavenly Palace, Celestial Storehouse)

Window to the Sky point

To open the spirit, one enters the middle palace (Zhongfu), passes through the cloud gate (Yuanmen), and accesses the inner palace (Tianfu) where the Creator of the soul, or God, resides and spiritual essence is stored. This is the point where we connect with our concept of God and the awe-inspiring natural world—it gives us security as it reminds us we are of the same essence. In this best palace, the spirit can be cleansed, fed, nurtured, and revitalized. This point is spiritually rejuvenating, raising the quality of essence. It is a psychologically revitalizing point and can be used to treat all emotional problems deriving from a lung disharmony, such as depression, confusion, forgetfulness, agoraphobia, and claustrophobia. It opens a person to a more meaningful existence by drawing them out of their shell, enhancing receptivity, communication, and trust. In the dying process, this allows the patient to let go of struggle, feelings of unfairness, and anger. It allows them to accept the dying process as a natural conclusion to the life cycle and to give up the illusion of control over that process. Physiologically, this point allows people to breathe more easily—treating asthma, epistaxis, and localized pain in the medial upper arm.

Lu 7 (Lieque) (Narrow Defile, Broken Sequence)

Exit point; Luo/Connecting point with Large Intestine; Xi/Confluent/Opening/Meeting point of the Ren/Conception Channel

Treating a patient with this point brings balance to all of the officials, so it can be used to treat almost everything. The corporeal soul resides in the lungs, so treating with this point releases emotional tensions. If a patient is suffering in silence, this point brings harmony and balance. For depression, frustration, and worry, or incompletely expressed grief or sadness, this point can help release tears or other forms of emotional expression. By treating repressed emotions, it calms the mind and resolves symptoms of anxiety, including restless sleep, tension in the shoulders, tightness or feelings of oppression in the chest, and shallow breathing. It is a good point for treating migraines, neck rigidity, and tension headaches and all facial conditions, including trigeminal neuralgia, lock jaw, toothaches, facial paralysis, and facial tics. It communicates with the large intestine channel to help with constipation. It clears and regulates the conception channel and benefits the bladder and opens water passages.

Lu 9 (Taiyuan) (Very Great/Greater Abyss)

Hui/Gathering/Meeting/Eight Influential point for Vessels; Mother/Reinforcing/Tonification point; Shu/Stream/Transporting point; Tu/Earth point; Yuan/Primary/Source point

This is a strong revival point for patients suffering from collapse, concussion, asphyxia, or poison. It promotes circulation by tonifying gathering qi to treat exhaustion, listlessness, cold extremities, and palpitations. If the patient is suffering from mental chaos, or doesn't have a regular pulse and you cannot make an adequate diagnosis due to arrhythmia, use this point first. Physically, this point tonifies lung yin and qi and resolves phlegm to treat asthma, shortness of breath on exertion, cough, fluid retention in the lungs and general edema, hemoptysis, indigestion, pain in the wrist or arm, and sore throat.

This point can also be used for spiritual chaos—when a patient feels as if life doesn't make sense and things are just "going to hell." During the dying process, this point revives the patient to allow them the clarity of thought and strength of body to help them make a smooth transition.

Large Intestine: Hand Yang Ming
LI 4 (Hegu) (Adjoining Valleys, Joining of the Valleys, Union Valley)

Entry point; Yuan/Source/Primary point

This is a great point for detoxifying the body and the mind. Known as the "great eliminator," it expels wind heat and releases the exterior—often relaxing muscular tension and giving the patient an emotional release, alleviating anxiety and powerfully calming the mind. For the dying patient, it promotes a smooth evolution into the dying process by allowing the patient to relax and let go.

Hegu stops pain and removes obstruction from the channel by harmonizing the ascending and descending and promoting an antispasmodic action which can be used for pain in the intestines or uterus. It treats inflammation or loss of function anywhere in the channel. It is an excellent point for increasing salivation and decreasing nausea, emesis, and loss of appetite. It increases the quality of life by increasing plasma leucine-enkephalin, thus stimulating the immune system and decreasing fatigue, dizziness, and weakness. This point tonifies qi and consolidates the exterior. It stimulates the dispersing function of the lungs, which resolves breathlessness.

LI 11 (Quchi) (Crooked Pond)

Mother/Reinforcing/Tonification point; He/Sea/Uniting point; Tu/Earth point

This point may be used for many different conditions as it influences both the exterior and the interior and has a wide range of actions. It cools heat, expels wind, and regulates the blood, so it may be used for hypertension as well as anemia. It resolves dampness and regulates nutritive qi and may be used to tonify the channel. It is used in painful arthritic conditions to benefit the joints and sinews.

LI 17 (Tianding) (Heaven's Vessel, Heavenly Vessel, Celestial Tripod)

In ancient China, a ding was a precious, sacrificial vessel. In this case, the head is the precious vessel because the brain is held within it. The original spirit resides in the storehouse of the brain. This point is one of the strongest on the Large Intestine/Colon Channel; it cleans the vessel by clearing the mind and spirit of toxins. Tian refers to the heavens; connecting to this point allows the patient to surrender the tendency to cling to life. It promotes relaxation and allows the patient to let go and have a smooth transition into the dying process. When the patient has a loss of voice or the voice is inhibited, this point can be used to clear throat and lung qi.

LI 18 (Futu) (Support the Prominence, Support and Rush Out, Protuberance Assistance)

Window to the Sky point

Like Tianding, Futu allows the patient to surrender the tendency to cling to life. It promotes relaxation and allows the patient to let go and have a smooth transition into the dying process. It also benefits the throat by relieving coughing, resolving phlegm, and dispersing masses, so it allows the patient to have a clearer voice. This is particularly true in relationships, as Futu is concerned with the expression and free flow of energy in human bonding. Futu means to aid or assist suddenly or abruptly. For patients who have suffered a loss or feel lonely and shut off, this point releases them from their self-imposed prison. It treats depression by dispersing dark and heavy thoughts and helps the patient to find pleasure of being alive moment by moment in the time they have left.

Water

Kidney: Foot Shao Yin
K 3 (Taixi) (Great Creek, Greater Mountain Stream, Great Ravine)

Shu/Stream/Transporting point; Tu/Earth point; Yuan/Primary/ Source point

The Earth point of a Water meridian, this is an important point for emotional stability, especially when a patient is dealing with life choices and coming from a place of fear. Tonifying this point can tap into the reserves of Water that allow a person to adapt to changes in a way that is quick and smooth-flowing. In stabilizing emotions, it calms the mind and balances the will so that a person can feel in control of their decision-making abilities. This point may be used when a patient looks weak-willed or emotionally labile, alternating periods of hyperactivity and anxiety with depression and inactivity. It can also be used for patients who are physically tired but restless, or patients who find life an effort, but are driven on by emotional restlessness and willpower. This point may be used for patients experiencing fearfulness, insomnia with frightening dreams, or who express that they are seeing everything as difficult and they are afraid to make decisions. Taixi benefits essence and strengthens the lower back and knees, and can be used to treat most genito-urinary disorders. This point goes straight to the core of original qi, and tonifies the kidneys in qi, jing, yin, and yang deficiency patterns. It is also used in palliative care to increase salivation for patients dealing with chronic dry mouth.

K 20 (Futonggu) (Connecting Valley on the Abdomen, Through the Valley, Open Valley, Rice Chong Valley)

Crossing/Coalescent/Point of Intersection with the Chong; Spirit point

The name of this point refers to the place on the abdomen where it is found. It eases feelings of negativity and is a spiritually peaceful place. Treating this valley evokes a feeling of a peaceful place, sheltered, fertile, and tranquil—a protected haven. It can be used for patients facing death with thoughts of loneliness or suicide. K 20 can be used to ease fear of being trapped and to give comfort and strength for dealing with darkness. It regulates channel qi, stops pain, and regulates stomach and intestine functions. Therefore, it is cleansing and moves waste products through.

K 21 (Youmen) (Secluded Door, Pylorus Gate, Dark Gate)

Crossing/Coalescent/Point of Intersection with the Chong; Spirit point

Youmen can be used to ease fear. It restores a sense of balance between work and rest, laughter and crying, night and day, dark and light. When everything appears dark, it helps to relive and resolve old issues where new light needs to be shed on them. This point is good for patients who are stuck feeling as if they are going through hell with no way out. If this gate is stuck closed, the person will experience a sort of mental torment where they cannot stop thinking negatively. Opening the gate allows the person to see that they can face their fears. It descends rebellious stomach qi to harmonize the stomach. This is the last point on the Kidney Channel to connect with the Chong Channel, so it may be used to regulate qi and blood.

K 23 (Shenfeng) (Spirit's Seal, Mind Seal, Spirit Envelops)

Spirit point

K 23, 24, and 25 are all big reservoirs of spirit and can be considered together and have similar functions—they all calm the mind by reducing anxiety and mental restlessness. Shenfeng calms and reconnects the spirit, regulates qi, and unblocks the collateral of the breasts. It eases fear and brings inner strength. This point can be used when a person cannot see or feel their identity, uniqueness, or integrity. For feelings of being disconnected or disempowered, this point brings the patient together when they are feeling fragmented. It tonifies the kidneys and calms the mind to relieve anxiety and mental restlessness deriving from kidney deficiency.

K 24 (Lingxu) (Spirit's Ruins, Spirit's Burial Ground, Spirit's Place)

Spirit point

Like Shenfeng, Lingxu is a big reservoir of spirit that calms anxiety and eases fear to promote a calm mind and inner strength. It is close to the heart where the spirit resides and its yin aspects are represented. It tonifies the kidneys to treat mental restlessness and insomnia caused by kidney deficiency. When a person appears lifeless, spiritless, with no life spark, or totally resigned, this is the best point on the body to bring back life and resuscitate the spirit. It restores a sense of the patient's true self. Physically, it unblocks collateral of the breasts and opens the chest to treat breathing difficulties, including shortness of breath, asthma, and coughing. It regulates qi to relieve vomiting and brings pleasure back to eating.

K 25 (Shencang) (Spirit's Storage, Storehouse)

Spirit point

This third spirit point is the reservoir to tap into when a person is feeling totally depleted and as if the well of life has run dry. In extreme deficiency, a patient may use up what energy they have as soon as they gain some. Patients may present as desperate, anxious, worried, fearful, sleepless, or in a deep mental rut, having lost all joy at being alive. Using this point can tap into the deep spring to gain new reserves and nourish the spirit. Opening the Storehouse tonifies the kidneys to resolve deficiency and brings calmness to the mind and spirit to build the patient's inner strength.

Urinary Bladder: Foot Tai Yang
UB 44 (39) (Shengtang) (Spirit's Hall, Mind Hall, Main House Facing South of Spirit)

Spirit point

This point is next to the back-transporting point of the heart. It can be used to calm the mind and resolve spiritual issues by keeping the gate of shen (spirit) open. It treats physical, emotional, and psychological problems related to the heart, including trauma, anxiety, palpitations, stuffy or oppressive feelings in the chest, cardiac pain, insomnia, and depression.

UB 47 (42) (Hunmen) (Door of the Ethereal Soul, Soul's Door, Gate of Soul)

Spirit point

This point is next to the back-transporting point of the liver and can be used for people presenting wooden qualities in their emotions— long-standing anger, resentment, frustration, and depression with no movement. This point roots the ethereal soul, thus allowing the patient to let go and open the gate to a grounded sense of direction or purpose for their life. For severely yin-deficient patients, it eases night fears. By supporting Wood and draining Water, it can be used to treat patients who are having difficulty eating or drinking; it stops vomiting and reduces chest, hypochondriac, and back pain. This is a good point for patients with a history of alcohol and/or drug abuse.

UB 52 (47) (Zhishi) (Will's Dwelling, Willpower Room, Memory Room)

Spirit point

This point is in line with the back-transporting point of the kidneys. If a patient is depressed and disoriented, reinforcing this point strengthens willpower and determination to lift the spirit. It gives the patient much-needed mental strength to make an effort to get better and overcome feelings of hopelessness. It tonifies the kidneys and strengthens the back in the kidney area to treat weakness from overworking, urinary problems, impotence, and menstrual irregularities.

UB 57 (Chengshan) (Support the Mountain, Supporting Mountain)

This point is used primarily to let go of fear. It invigorates the blood, relaxes the sinews, clears heat, and is used as a distal point for treating lower back pain and sciatica. This point regulates qi in the yang organs and removes obstructions from the channels. It is an empirical point for treating hemorrhoids.

UB 61 (Pucan/Pushen) (Serve and Consult, Servant's Aide, Kowtow, Kiss Master's Foot)

Crossing/Coalescent/Points of Intersection with Yangwei and Yangqiao Channels

Pucan helps patients to regain the ability to stand up on their own, to face and let go of their fears. This is an excellent point to treat leg cramps, muscular atrophy, weakness of the lower extremities, and heel pain.

UB 64 (Jinggu) (Capital Bone)

Yuan/Primary/Source point

Jinggu helps patients to get back on their feet by letting go of fear. It disperses and eliminates wind and clears the brain to calm the mind and spirit. This point can be used to treat headaches, blurred vision, and epilepsy. It clears heat and strengthens the back and can be used to treat excessive pain in chronic backaches.

Other points

The following points are not traditional Five Element points but have powerful effects on hospice patients.

Governor: Du
Du (GV) 20 (Baihui) (Hundred Meetings, One Hundred Meetings)

> Ancestor point; Crossing/Coalescent/Point of Intersection with Urinary Bladder Channel; Crossing/Meeting point of All Yang Channels; Sea of Marrow point

This is a very important point for hospice patients. It is considered to be the opening of the crown chakra on the physical body, and thus it is the place where the soul leaves the body. It is a well point and the place where the energy flow in the body changes direction. All six yang channels meet the Governing Channel here. This point can be used to pull the fragmented person back together by accessing the wisdom of the ancestors. By moving a person forward and clearing the senses, it helps patients gain a different level of understanding, connecting with departed loved ones and to the saints, sages, and sacred beings with whom they identify. It clears the mind and lifts the spirit. It brings a sense of peace, comfort, and stability in times of agitation or depletion, but should not be used if the patient is in acute distress.

This point can be used to treat prolapsed qi, yang, and/or organs. Mental problems, including depression, apathy, exhaustion, nervous tension, restlessness, insomnia, feelings of vulnerability and hurt, mania, giddiness, frightful palpitations, and deathlike inversions, may be treated by either tonifying for deficient conditions or reducing in excess conditions.

Baihui treats many physical conditions. If a patient loses consciousness during an acupuncture treatment, Du/GV 20 (Baihui) promotes resuscitation. It is widely used in palliative care to increase salivation in patients suffering from dry mouth (xerostomia). It may also be used to treat stiff necks, headaches, hypertension, visual disturbances, dizziness, tetany, wind stroke, and chronic diarrhea.

Conception: Ren
Ren (CV) 14 (Juque) (Great Palace, Great Deficiency, Great Tower Gate)

Mu/Front/Collecting point of the Heart

This is a potent point to calm the spirit by directly connecting the patient to the heart, the seat of shen. It keeps the gate of shen open, supplying energy to the mind, body, and spirit. It clears the heart and calms the mind. It eases fear, soothes the chest, slows the heart, and transforms phlegm to treat tremendous confusion, raving, manic rage, addictions, and nervous exhaustion with over-enthusiasm and anxiety. It allows the supreme controller to come back to power.

Juque pacifies the stomach by subduing rebellious stomach qi and can be used to treat digestive problems of an emotional origin. It benefits the diaphragm and can be used in panic attacks.

Extra points
Sishencong (Four Mind Hearing, Four Spirits, Four Intelligences)
The four points of Sishencong are effective treatment points for headaches, insomnia, poor memory, and vertigo. These points subdue interior wind to treat dizziness, blurred vision, epilepsy, and "madness" characterized by hallucinations caused by prolonged depression and anger.

Chapter 9

The Major Hospice Diagnoses

The remainder of this book includes a detailed list defining the major hospice diagnoses and related signs and symptoms. It examines primary and adjunct TCM and Asian Medicine treatments for palliative care. While it is not exhaustive, it does confirm that acupuncture has a place in hospice and palliative care. It discusses and encourages further research areas and clinical applications for both current findings and future studies.

Let's move beyond the broader definitions of life-limiting illness and terminal illness to the practical application of information to find out what makes a specific hospice diagnosis. There are general guidelines for determining a person's eligibility for hospice care. As we have reviewed previously, the Palliative Performance Scale (PPS) is one tool that is used extensively. Criteria for hospice care include being dependent on someone else for at least two activities of daily living, scoring 70 percent or less on the PPS, now in its second version, the PPSv2 (Fox 2010), and specific criteria for each of the general diagnoses (usually based on abnormal laboratory values, and/or decreases in function, and/or a combination of measurable signs and symptoms) (Hospice by the Bay 2018).

What are the major hospice diagnoses?

Currently, there are only ten major hospice diagnoses. Nine are based on specific disease categories, but anyone who is expected to die in the next six months may be admitted by their doctor, if they are hospice eligible or hospice appropriate. These categories are limited, often by insurance companies, but there is some room for broader interpretations. They are:

1. Cancer

2. Dementia

3. Heart disease

4. HIV/AIDS

5. Liver disease

6. Neurological disease

7. Pulmonary disease

8. Renal failure

9. Stroke or coma

10. Terminal illness: general (non-specific).

For each hospice diagnosis, we will look at a general definition of the disease and the criteria for admission to a hospice. After the criteria section, you will find an information section related to the diagnosis, and some patient profiles to help provide an overview of the disease process. Next there will be acupuncture research topics, and some directed treatment for relief of symptoms, or other means of improving patient comfort.

Cancer

Cancer is a group of diseases involving abnormal cell growth with the potential to invade or spread to other parts of the body.

Hospice criteria for cancer

- Clinical finding of malignancy with widespread aggressive or progressive disease as evidenced by increasing symptoms worsening lab values and/or evidence of metastatic disease.

- PPS < 70 percent.

- Patient refuses further life-prolonging therapy OR continues to decline in spite of definitive therapy.

- Supporting documentation of hypercalcemia > 12 (hypercalcemia is a condition in which the calcium level in your blood is above normal. Too much calcium in your blood can weaken your bones, create kidney stones, and interfere with how your heart and brain work. Hypercalcemia is usually a result of overactive parathyroid glands)

- Cachexia with a weight loss of 5 percent of total body weight in the past three months.

- Recurrent disease after surgery/radiation/chemotherapy.

- Signs and symptoms of advanced disease, including but not limited to nausea, requirement of transfusions, malignant ascites, or pleural effusion.

Comorbid or secondary conditions:

- Chronic obstructive pulmonary disease

- Congestive heart failure

- Liver disease

- Alcoholism

- Renal failure

- Dementia

- Neurological disease.

More information on cancer

In the not too distant past, a cancer diagnosis was considered a death sentence. New discoveries about the nature of cancer cells, and new medications for the treatment of some forms of cancer, have changed that prognosis from dying to cured. The treatment philosophy for many types of cancers for years was to try to fool the cancer cell by attacking it from the outside. In the past few years, this approach has been modified, and newer treatments are geared toward modifying the patient's own immune system to turn off or destroy the cancer cell. Even with billions of dollars in research, new medications, the most advanced diagnostic tools, and approaches to combat the mutation of cells, cancer is still the number one cause of death in the US and many other parts of the world.

Why is cancer so hard to treat? It is often missed. The first thing to understand is that there are over 100 kinds of cancer. They don't all look or act the same. Some are genetic, while others are triggered by environmental (exogenous) pathogens or conditions. Some are fast growing, some are slower and less life threatening. There are cancers that can be cured by surgery, radiation, or chemotherapy, or a combination of those techniques. More aggressive cancers do not respond to treatments. Oncology is a vast field, and the field of medicine where acupuncturists are called on most often to help in patient care, simply for one reason—the patients demanded it.

In 2018, it is estimated that 9.6 million people died from cancer (World Health Organization 2018b). The **most common causes of cancer death** worldwide are:

- Lung (1.76 million deaths)

- Colorectal (862,000 deaths)

- Stomach (783,000 deaths)

- Liver (782,000 deaths)

- Breast (627,000 deaths).

Skin and prostate cancer are the next most common forms of cancer. Another reason cancer is so deadly is the disease's presentation. In many cases, the growth is internalized. Cancer may not cause pain in the body until the later stages when a tumor or multiple tumors start to affect the organs, or grow to press against a vein or a nerve. Some forms of cancer prevention rely on people completing self-exams (i.e. testicular and breast cancer). Often the cancer has grown and then metastasized (spread) to other organs before the patient experiences any clinical symptoms. This pattern of growth has caused many people to believe that cancer killed someone quickly, when the truth of the matter is, they may have been living with the disease for years.

A final piece of the puzzle belongs to healthcare systems and over-population. The current system of medicine is not based on the most effective and humane care of an individual. Instead, doctor visits are based on cost-effective care, which focuses on seeing the maximum number of patients in the minimum amount of time. Imagine if the above patient visited a very busy doctor's office, when her complaint was only of a cough. If the patient appears otherwise normal, some physicians may not even listen to the complete lung fields. They may not order a chest x-ray, or they may ask the patient if they want a chest x-ray. They may, after spending less than five minutes with the patient, simply write a prescription for an antibiotic or a cough syrup, and send the patient home. The next doctor they see may be the one who finds the cancer.

In some countries, care is based on what will be covered under a patient's insurance, which dictates or limits certain tests and procedures. It is a system in which many physicians have stated they feel their hands are tied. They have been rewarded for increasing corporate profits and spending less time per patient. Instead of practicing medicine and honing their diagnostic skills, many doctors feel they have been forced to leave the diagnosis to machines and laboratory work, and treatment more often than not is in the form of a prescription medication, with no time for patient education on prevention.

Examples of patients

Patients may not know what to expect, or may have symptoms that look like another disease. For example, Patient C, who generally feels healthy and is active, suddenly becomes weak, and loses her appetite. She develops a cough that she thought was from hay fever, but it is persistent, and worsens. Her voice is hoarse. Finally, she goes to the hospital because she is having difficulty breathing, and believes she has bronchitis or the flu.

On examination, the doctor hears abnormal lung sounds on one side of the patient's body. The rales and rhonchi make her suspect that the woman has pneumonia. She orders a chest x-ray, and the results come back showing black spots on the lower lobe of the lung. Next, the doctor orders blood work which shows liver function abnormalities, and a CT scan that reveals tumors on the lungs and the upper margin of the liver. At this point, it is clear that the patient has Stage IV cancer with multiple organ involvement. Cancer is staged by the level of cancerous cells found in the body. Stage 0 means there's no cancer, only abnormal cells with the potential to become cancer. In Stage I the cancer is small and only in one area. Stages II and III mean the cancer is larger and has grown into nearby tissues or lymph nodes. Stage IV means the cancer has spread to other parts of your body (DerSarkissian 2019). The hospice criteria for terminal cancer, generally, is reserved for patients with Stage IV.

Even with this information, the patient's health is declining so rapidly she is discharged from the hospital directly into hospice care, where she dies eight days after admission. This woman is 92 years old, so while the family is shocked by this loss, they are able to rationalize that she had a good, long life and that death at this age is a normal, natural conclusion. The family of someone of such advanced age has most likely discussed what kind of care she might need if she became infirm. They would probably know if she had completed advanced directives, or had a funeral plan, and at the very least, they would understand she was near to the end of her lifespan.

Now, imagine if the patient was a 57-year-old with two sets of children from two marriages, and the family's primary wage earner, who didn't have a clear will. Things get much more complicated. This is not to suggest that one family's grief is more difficult than another's, but an unexpected death is just the beginning of the consequences of that loss.

We often foster an idea that everyone gets to live a good, long life, but that isn't always the case. If we hold on to that belief, then we never make plans to deal with our own death and its repercussions. Perhaps this lack of planning stems from a fear of immortality, but the results can be calamitous for the survivors. Unfortunately, thousands of people die every day around the world. This is why, in a hospice, the family of the patient is also considered the patient. Survivors are offered grief counseling and other related services after the primary patient dies.

Acupuncture research and role in cancer care

How can acupuncture help with cancer patients? We can spend more time with patient care, do complete physical examinations, treat the root of the problem, as well as their symptoms, and refer to specialists.

Older studies have shown clinically significant treatment outcomes for treating symptoms of cancer with acupuncture. One example of this is a 2013 *Current Oncology* article which proved 333 lung cancer patients showed statistically significant improvements in pain levels and appetite, decreased nausea and nervousness, and overall improvement in well-being after receiving treatments one to two times per week for 45 minutes. The acupuncture points used were LI 4 (Hegu), Liv 3 (Taichong), St 36 (Zusanli), Sp 6 (Sanyinjiao), and Lu 7 (Lieque). It should be noted here that these are all points already discussed in the Hospice Acupuncture Protocol. The points listed above were enhanced with auricular acupuncture on Shenmen, Subcortex, and Zero. More importantly, the subjects showed no significant side effects from the treatment (Kasymjanova *et al.* 2013).

Unfortunately, many studies offer good information, but are presented in an unacceptable form. In a systematic review of acupuncture in cancer care and a synthesis of the evidence (Garcia *et al.* 2013), the authors screened 2151 publications but found that only 41 RCTs (randomized controlled trials) involving eight symptoms (pain, nausea, hot flashes, fatigue, radiation-induced xerostomia, prolonged postoperative ileus, anxiety/mood disorders, and sleep disturbance) met all inclusion criteria. According to the review, 33 of those studies had a high risk of bias. After their exhaustive review, the authors concluded that acupuncture is an appropriate adjunctive treatment for chemotherapy-induced nausea/vomiting, but additional studies are needed.

For acupuncturists who are now conducting research, or are considering becoming researchers, the reviewers of RCTs generously offered the following expert advice: To fulfill scientifically based medical criteria, further acupuncture research should focus on standardizing comparison groups and treatment methods, be at least single-blinded studies, assess biologic mechanisms, have adequate statistical power, and involve multiple acupuncturists (Garcia *et al.* 2013). We have thousands of years of practice behind our medicine, but we aren't getting the insurance companies to pay for us because we do not have enough scientifically based, statistically significant, or technical correct data to prove that we can duplicate our results, and because our practice models lean heavily toward single practitioners who do not collaborate with colleagues.

What does Asian Medicine do differently?

We know that, if you bring the body back into balance, it strengthens the immune system, and there are new treatments for cancer that focus on actually turning the body's immune system back on. This may be one chasm where we are now working on the same bridge. Allopathic medicine traditionally looked for one solution for all patients, for instance chemotherapy for all cancer patients; Asian Medicine was looking at the individual patient as a unique entity with many possible solutions for a disharmony. The latest trend in allopathy is to individualize treatments based on a person's DNA, which may give all forms of medicine more treatment choices.

We've discussed the hospice criteria, but there are also ten common symptoms of cancer that have been proposed: pain, nausea/vomiting, loss of appetite, constipation, fever, diarrhea, bloating, pressure ulcers, depression/anxiety, and sleep disorders. It should be noted that from the TCM perspective, one could argue nausea is not the same as vomiting, nor is depression the same as anxiety. Alternatively, 36 common symptoms of cancer have been categorized: infection, difficulty swallowing, nausea/vomiting, anorexia, dry mouth, constipation, diarrhea, intestinal obstruction, ascites, malnutrition, coughing, breathing difficulties, hiccoughs, flu-like syndrome, urinary tract infection, urinary incontinence, headache, anxiety, insomnia, delirium, convulsions, anxiety, depression, thrombosis, disseminated intravascular coagulation (a condition in which blood clots form throughout the body, blocking small blood vessels), anemia, edema, hypercalcemia, spasms, pimple rash, fatigue, muscle atrophy, thrush, massive bleeding, acute pain, and suffocation.

Common symptoms of cancer are classified into the following diseases according to TCM classifications: loss of consciousness, convulsions, blood syndromes, cough, asthma disease, pleural fluid retention, vomiting, hiccoughs, dysphagia occlusion, constipation, diarrhea, mouth sores, strangury disease, urinary incontinence, palpitations, insomnia, coma, abdominal retention, headache, consumptive disease, edema, and fever due to internal injuries. The classifications differed slightly among different ancient Chinese physicians. For instance, Li Yan divided the common symptoms into 41 types for pattern identification. His detailed descriptions for these symptoms were highly informative for clinical practices. Identification and treatment of the major symptoms are essential components, as is the basis of pattern identification.

The research for this book uncovered many papers on the effects of acupuncture. Many were insightful, but not helpful because they were highly generalized. For instance, radiotherapy (radiation) has a frequently seen side effect of dry mouth. In one study, the patients were treated with LI 1 (Shangyang), Lu 7 (Lieque), St 36 (Zusanli), and Ren/CV 24 (Chengjiang); and auricular points Shenmen, Salivary Gland 2, and Point Zero. While it was true that the patients saw significant improvements with weekly treatment, there were only two of them in this study. The patients' SXI (Summated Xerostomia Index) scores declined from a maximum possible score of 60 (a score of 0 indicated no dry mouth) for the respective weeks of treatment as follows: Patient 1's scores were 30, 23, 21, 12, 6, and 7; Patient 2's scores were 34, 23, 11, and 10.

Does this mean you should not try treating your patients who are experiencing xerostomia with these points? No. Is this a scientifically significant result? No. Do you think if the patient got good relief without added side effects that they would care? Could you prove this scientifically by creating a double-blind study with other acupuncturists? Yes. As a historical point of accuracy, many studies from China did not include the use of placebos or sham acupuncture points because they believed it was unethical to withhold proper treatment for patients who were suffering. The scientific model is a relative newcomer to medicine, often funded by large pharmaceutical companies which have been known at times to produce the most profitable drugs but not always the best medicines available.

One study (Deng *et al.* 2007) monitored women who were experiencing facial flashes (hot flashes) after starting antiestrogen therapy for breast cancer. They underwent four weeks of treatment with three acupuncture sessions per week. Vital signs, including blood pressure, pulse rate, and body temperature, were measured before treatment. The treatments lasted 20–25 minutes. Acupuncture was performed by a Traditional Korean Medicine (TKM) physician who had at least three years of clinical experience in acupuncture treatment. Acupuncture points were selected according to the recommendations of TKM clinical experts and standard acupuncture textbooks.

Five points—Du/GV 20 (Baihui); M-HN-3 (Yintang); and bilaterally at H 8 (Shaofu), K 10 (Yingu), and Liv 2 (Xingjian)— were chosen. Needles were gently manipulated manually to obtain de qi (needle sensation referring to pain, numbness, and distension felt around the point after the needle is inserted to a certain depth as well as the operator's sensation of tension around the needle). After ten minutes, the needles were gently rotated without evoking de qi. The findings suggest that acupuncture is a useful alternative treatment for alleviating facial flashes in patients with breast cancer who are undergoing antiestrogen therapy.

Another study (Kanakura *et al.* 2002) measured the effectiveness of acupuncture and moxibustion treatments on lymphedema following intrapelvic lymph node dissection. Twelve patients undergoing intrapelvic lymph node dissection for carcinoma of the uterine cervix, carcinoma of the uterine body, or for ovarian cancer were entered into the study. Patients receiving radiation therapy were excluded.

The following acupuncture points were chosen for treatment of lymphedema: St 36 (Zusanli), Sp 6 (Sanyinjiao), UB 23 (Shenshu),

UB 67 (Zhiyin), K 1 (Yongquan), Ren/CV 2 (Qugu), Ren/CV 3 (Zhongji), and Ren/CV 12 (Zhongwan). Moxa sticks were used for UB 67 (Zhiyin) and Kyuto-shin for other points. Kyuto-shin is a method that potentiates the effects of both moxibustion and acupuncture by placing and burning moxa on the head of the needle. Patient sessions lasted 15–20 minutes and were given five times per week during hospitalization and twice per week at the outpatient clinic.

In cases 3, 6–9, 11, and 12, the patients had relatively mild edema. Their edema disappeared subjectively and objectively by two months after the start of treatments.

Cases 1, 2, 4, 5, 8, and 10 showed marked improvement. Their hardened and swollen lower extremities gradually softened in all patients at two to three weeks after the start of treatment. Edema began to disappear at the same time. However, a subjectively and objectively satisfactory recovery required four months or more in all patients.

Case 1 was complicated not only with lymphedema of the lower extremities, but also with lymph cysts in the inguinal region and pelvis. Lymphedema and lymph cysts could be eliminated during a period of more than one year, in which punctures and aspirations were repeatedly performed, in addition to persevering with acupuncture and moxibustion treatments.

From these results, it was confirmed that acupuncture and moxibustion have therapeutic and preventive effects on lymphedema, and should be integrated into Western medicine to improve the patient's quality of life.

Fever due to impairment of internal organs often occurs in cancer patients. The following information is an excerpt from a paper on differentiation and herbal recommendations for fevers (Hopkins Technology 1995).

Fever of functional and unknown origins and that occurring with tumors, blood diseases, tuberculosis, endocrine diseases, diseases of connective tissue and some chronic infectious diseases may be differentiated and treated with the principles mentioned in this section.

Differentiation between asthenia and sthenia syndromes: In the development of diseases, asthenia of healthy qi and sthenia of pathogenic factors oppose each other and are also related to each other. Therefore, asthenia syndrome and sthenia syndrome may appear simultaneously or transform into each other and appear in sequence. At the critical stage of diseases, there may appear false sthenia and false asthenia manifestations. Fever due to impairment of internal organs mostly manifests itself as asthenia-syndrome, but whether qi or blood, yin or yang, is predominantly deficient and which Zang-organ is involved should be determined. In cases with sthenia-syndrome, it should be differentiated whether qi stagnation or blood stasis is present.

For fever due to yin deficiency, give Modified Powder for Clearing Away Heat from Bone.

The formula for fever due to blood deficiency is The Modified Decoction of Invigorating the Spleen and Nourishing the Heart.

If the fever is due to Qi deficiency, The Modified Decoction for Strengthening the Middle Jiao and Benefiting Qi is given.

For fever due to Yang Deficiency, prescribe the Modified Pill for Invigorating Kidney-Qi.

With fever due to stagnated liver-qi, the recommended formula is a modification of Xiaoyao Powder of Moutan Radicis and Gardeniae.

And finally, if the fever is due to blood stasis, use The Modified Decoction for Removing Blood Stasis in the Chest.

While it is beyond the scope of this book to discuss treatments for every kind of cancer, it is important to note that acupuncture does have a place in helping to recognize subclinical signs of imbalance. Part of educating patients and other professionals is that we must also fight against incorrect assumptions. The article "Replacing conventional medicine for complementary therapy can decrease survival" (Therrien 2018) is a perfect example of misleading information.

It stated that people who received complementary therapy for curable cancers were more likely to refuse at least one component of their conventional cancer treatment, and were more likely to die as a result, according to researchers from Yale Cancer Center. The researchers compared 258 patients who used complementary medicine to 1032 who did not. Researchers linked the lower chances of survival to refusing or delaying standard treatments. The study did not include data on the exact therapies people used, but lead author, Dr. Skyler Johnson, from Yale School of Medicine, noted they were more likely to be alternative medicines—rather than complementary therapies like yoga or massage, which are usually used alongside standard treatments. By collecting the outcomes of patients who did receive complementary medicine in addition to conventional cancer treatments, the researchers found a greater risk of death.

Despite having received some conventional cancer therapy, these patients were more likely to refuse other aspects of recommended care like chemotherapy, surgery, radiation, and/or hormone therapy. Conversely, Matin Ledwick, Cancer Research UK's head information nurse, said complementary medicine might help improve well-being or quality of life for some patients.

Professor Arnie Purushotham, director at King's Health Partners Comprehensive Cancer Centre, said:

> There was a clear difference between alternative therapies and complementary treatments. However, there is increasing evidence that complementary therapy like acupuncture, yoga, and relaxation therapy may be beneficial in alleviating cancer patients' symptoms like pain and fatigue. (Therrien 2018)

One could easily argue that the writer of the article did not delve deeply into the scientific research studies that have proven acupuncture is effective for cancer patients and has been utilized for much more than fatigue and pain relief. The article is also quite vague about what forms of "complementary medicines" he is referring too. Sadly, laypeople frequently use the terms complementary and alternative medicine interchangeably, which means the title of his article could bolster a bias against Asian Medicine.

Dementia

Dementia is a general term for a decline in mental ability severe enough to interfere with daily life. Dementia includes Alzheimer's disease (AD), also called senile dementia, and Lewy body dementia. AD is the most common type of dementia. Short-term memory loss is the most common symptom during early onset.

Hospice criteria for dementia

1. Stage 7c or beyond on the Functional Assessment Staging Test (FAST) (see Table 9.1) (Reisberg 1988). FAST is the most validated measure of the course of AD in published, scientific literature. Use the FAST tool to determine if changes in a patient's condition are due to Alzheimer's disease or another condition. If the patient's changes are due to AD progression, then their changes will follow the sequence of FAST. AD-related changes do not skip FAST stages, but other forms of dementia may skip stages.

Table 9.1: The Functional Assessment Staging Test (FAST)

Stage	Stage name	Characteristics	Expected untreated AD duration	Mental age (years)	MMSE score
1	Normal	No deficiencies		Adult	29–30
2	Possible mild cognitive impairment	Subjective functional deficit			28–29
3	Mild cognitive impairment	Objective functional deficit interferes with a person's most complex task	84	12+	24–28
4	Mild dementia	IADLs become affected, such as bill paying, cooking, cleaning, traveling	24	8–12	19–20

5	Moderate dementia	Needs help selecting proper attire	18	5–7	15
6a	Moderately severe dementia	Needs help putting on clothes	4.8	5	9
6b	Moderately severe dementia	Needs help bathing	4.8	4	5
6c	Moderately severe dementia	Needs help toileting	4.8	4	5
6d	Moderately severe	Urinary incontinence	3.6	3–4	3
6e	Moderately severe dementia	Fecal incontinence	9.6	2–3	1
7a	Severe dementia	Speaks five to six words during day	12	1–2.5	0
7b	Severe dementia	Speaks only one word clearly	18	1	0
7c	Severe dementia	Can no longer walk	12	1	0
7d	Severe dementia	Can no longer sit up	12	0.5–0.8	0
7e	Severe dementia	Can no longer smile	18	0.2–0.4	0
7f	Severe dementia	Can no longer hold up head	12+	0–0.2	0

2. Presence of comorbid disease distinct from the terminal illness will impact functional impairment. The combined effects of Alzheimer's and any comorbid condition should support a prognosis of six months or less. These conditions include:

- Chronic obstructive pulmonary disease

- Congestive heart failure

- Cancer

- Liver disease

- Renal failure

- Neurological disease.

3. Patients should have had one of the following secondary conditions within the past 12 months:

- Delirium

- Recurrent or intractable infections, such as pneumonia or other URI (upper respiratory infection)

- Pyelonephritis or another type of urinary tract infection

- Septicemia

- Decubitus ulcers, multiple, stage 3–4

- Fever, recurrent after antibiotics

- Inability to maintain sufficient fluid and calorie intake demonstrated by either of the following: 10 percent weight loss during the previous six months OR Serum albumin < 2.5gm/dl

- Aspiration pneumonia.

More information on dementia

Dementia is part of a group of disorders, and there are numerous causes. Often the picture that comes to mind when we talk about dementia is an older person who has become more and more forgetful. Changes in short-term memory or the ability to concentrate are considered early warning signs. Caregivers can be confused by fluctuations in a person's mental clarity if the long-term memory remains intact during the early stages of the disease process. Some partners report that the patient's day-to-day, or hour-to-hour, variances in clear thinking lead them to believe their partner was faking or exaggerating their memory loss.

Is dementia a life-limiting or terminal illness, or just an inconvenience? To illustrate the difference, there is a saying, "It is one thing to forget where you put your car keys, but another when you forget what they are used for." It is a problem that can have an effect on all aspects of a person's life.

Like cancer, there are several different kinds of dementia, with different biological causes. Some progress fast and some slow. A person can have a temporary form from a thyroid or vitamin imbalance or a partially reversible form of vascular dementia, after a stroke or a transient ischemic attack (TIA), but those are not terminal. In the early stages of most forms of dementia, the patient is forgetful but is still able to carry out activities of daily living.

Lewy body dementia is the second most common form of dementia. It is an umbrella term that includes Parkinson's disease dementia and dementia with Lewy bodies. Both forms are characterized by abnormal deposits of the protein alpha-synuclein in the brain. People with Lewy body dementia may experience visual hallucinations and changes in alertness and attention. Other effects include Parkinson's disease-like signs and symptoms such as rigid muscles, slow movement, and tremors. It is not uncommon for patients to experience difficulty sleeping or concentrating, and emotional issues such as apathy or depression.

Alzheimer's disease can take four to eight years from the early onset to the end of life. Again, this assumes that the "normal patient," under "normal conditions," will conform very neatly to the FAST chart. There are always exceptions, and extenuating circumstances, that do not fall neatly in these parameters. New medications are available to slow the progress of the symptoms, and some people have lived as long as 20 years with the disease. Alzheimer's has been nicknamed "The long goodbye." In the most aggressive forms of dementia, the patient progressively regresses into an infant-like state, in which they are unable to feed, clothe, bathe, or toilet themselves.

Patient profile

How is it that a 76-year-old patient may not remember what he had for breakfast, or even if he had breakfast, but on the same day, he may still be capable of sitting down and completing the Sunday version of the *New York Times* crossword puzzle? Three words: deep neural grooves. He started working on the crossword every Sunday with his father when he was 14, and continued that weekly practice throughout his life. Sixty-two years of analyzing clues and solving word problems created a deep neural groove that makes this part of his brain easy to access. Although he has had 72 years of daily breakfasts, that event's time, place, and ingredients are variable and happened just a couple of hours ago. It is processed by a different part of the brain.

What if you had a patient who was highly functional, but not oriented to place? For instance, Lola is a 73-year-old female who enjoyed a 20-year career as a pharmaceutical representative, and traveled extensively for her job. She is able to feed and clothe herself, but she forgets she is in an assisted living facility. She wakes up in a strange bed and assumes she is in a hotel. She can still carry on a conversation, and follow instructions, and it does not seem strange to her that she does not know the other people in her facility.

She has a problem with her bladder due to a mild stroke, and cannot empty it completely. She cannot wear a catheter, because she forgets it is in, and what it is for, and has a history of attempting to forcibly remove the tubing from her urethra. She has to be catharized every other day, which puts her at high risk of a urinary tract infection (UTI).

If a patient has a UTI, they can easily become confused, agitated, or incontinent. If you rated them by the FAST chart they might appear to fit the criteria for a rating of 6d. Once the infection is cleared up, they might truly be at 4. It is essential with dementia patients that you know your patient well, and also discuss what has been observed with their primary caregiver, as a sudden change is not always due to the primary disease process.

Dementia patients are often unreliable historians. Memory loss can be embarrassing, so they may answer what they think is correct for a question, or use generalized language if they simply don't know the truth, or cannot remember the correct answer. For instance, a patient might be asked, what did you have for breakfast today? The patient may not be able to recall, but when pressed, they might reply, "Oh, the usual I guess." Or they might say, "Oatmeal," but in truth they had eggs.

Gathering a history may have an added complication if the primary caregiver is a spouse or partner who also has some short-term memory loss. When working with dementia patients, it is best to ask questions in the simplest form possible, and wait for the person to respond before asking another question. The same is true if you need to give instructions—keep them short, simple, and singular, and wait patiently for the patient's response.

Acupuncture research for dementia

What do we know about acupuncture and Alzheimer's disease? In one animal-based study, acupuncture was applied to acupoints Du 20 (Baihui) and UB 23 (Shenshu) on laboratory rats with (drug) induced AD. Rats treated with electroacupuncture had a preserved structure of the brain, the hippocampus. The researcher noted that neuronal cell injury was markedly reduced as a result of acupuncture (Health CMi 2015).

The traditional function of Du/GV 20 (Baihui—Hundred Meetings) is to clear the senses and calm the spirit. It is also the point of intersection for the Du/GV and Bladder channel. UB 23 (Shenshu), is the Back-shu point of the kidney. Tonifying this point can strongly root the energy of the body. An energetically rooted body can balance psychological distress more easily, so UB 23 can treat anxiety and depression. Chronic depression has been strongly correlated with increased risk for Alzheimer's.

Scientific investigations with humans confirmed the animal-based results. Magnetic resonance imaging (MRI) demonstrated that acupuncture enhances brain activity in AD patients. After acupuncture, MRI revealed that AD patients had significant improvements in connectivity for both frontal and lateral regions of the hippocampus. It was noted that due to the cognitive impairment associated with AD, acupuncture on specific acupoints could modulate the cerebral blood flow and strengthen the hippocampal connectivity in AD patients (Health CMi 2015).

In dementia, as in most disease processes, it is best to start treatment in the earlier stages. Other considerations for treatment are the patient's comorbidities. Utilize a point selection that will treat more than one condition. The greatest positive effect with the least number of needles is the best strategy when working with people who can present with restlessness or mental agitation.

It is interesting to note that some of the secondary conditions, namely high or tidal fevers and delirium, are symptoms associated with the external course of the Leg Yang Brightness Stomach Channel. This is noteworthy from the scientific perspective of neurogastroenterology, which has discovered that there are more neurons in the gut than in either the spinal or the peripheral nervous system. Since a large percentage of neurotransmitter production happens in the alimentary canal, it is not too much of a stretch to think that treating the function of the stomach channel may affect the production of neurotransmitters found in the gut, such as norepinephrine, epinephrine, dopamine, and serotonin, and therefore be useful in treating dementia symptoms.

The new points may be helpful in the treatment of dementia as well. For example, a major indication for N-HN-23 (Xingfen) is "excitement" idiocy resulting from brain disease; N-HN-31 (Tounie) (Temple) is used for progressive loss of memory; and N-HN-51 (Zhinao #1–5) (Heal brain #1–5) has brain diseases as its only indication. These are experiential indications without added randomized controlled studies to prove their repeatable results, but patients have experienced relief previously. The new points and the neurotransmitter production levels related to Parkinsonism or other forms of dementia could make excellent research studies.

Heart disease

Heart disease or cardiovascular disease generally refers to conditions that involve narrowed or blocked blood vessels that can lead to a heart attack, chest pain (angina), or stroke. Other heart conditions, such as those that affect your heart's muscle, valves, or rhythm, are also considered forms of heart disease.

Hospice criteria for heart disease

To meet the hospice heart disease criteria, a patient will have 1 and either 2 or 3 in the following:

1. Congestive heart failure (CHF) with New York Heart Association (NYHA) Class IV symptoms and both significant symptoms at rest and inability to carry out even minimal physical activity without dyspnea or angina.

2. Is optimally treated (i.e. diuretics, vasodilators, angiotensin-converting-enzyme (ACE) inhibitor, or hydralazine and nitrates).

3. Angina pectoris at rest, resistant to standard nitrate therapy, and the patient is either not a candidate for/or has declined invasive procedures.

Supporting documentation includes:

- Ejection fraction (EF) < 20 percent

- Treatment-resistant systematic dysrhythmias

- History of cardiac-related syncope

- Cardiovascular accident (CVA) 2/2 cardiac embolism

- History of cardiac resuscitation

- Concomitant HIV disease.

More information on heart disease

To understand the hospice criteria for a diagnosis of heart disease, you must understand that symptoms are ranked by the NYHA Classes (adapted from Dogin and New York Heart Association, Criteria Committee 1994).

There are four levels of symptoms (IV is the worst):

- I. Is cardiac disease without other symptoms.

- II. Mild symptoms (shortness of breath or angina) and slight limitation during ordinary activity.

- III. Marked limitation in activity due to symptoms, even during ordinary activity, for example walking short distances (20–100m), comfortable only at rest.

- IV. Significant symptoms at rest. Inability to carry out even minimal physical activity without dyspnea or angina, and worsening of symptoms.

Likewise, it is good to know the following basic categories of heart medications, and what they do:

- Anticoagulants

- Antiplatelet agents and dual antiplatelet therapy

- ACE inhibitors

- Angiotensin II receptor blockers

- Angiotensin-receptor neprilysin inhibitors

- Beta blockers

- Calcium channel blockers

- Cholesterol-lowering medications

- Digitalis preparations

- Diuretics

- Vasodilators.

Another piece in the puzzle is ejection fraction (EF), a measurement, expressed as a percentage, of how much blood the left ventricle pumps out with each contraction. The normal range is between 50 and 70 percent, with 41–49 percent being borderline. An ejection fraction measurement higher than 75 percent may indicate a heart condition such as hypertrophic cardiomyopathy.

It should be noted that a patient can have a normal ejection fraction measurement and still have heart failure (called HFpEF or heart failure with preserved ejection fraction). If the heart muscle has become so thick and stiff that the ventricle holds a smaller than usual volume of blood, it might still seem to pump out a normal percentage of the blood that enters it. In reality, though, the total volume of blood ejected isn't enough to meet the body's needs.

Patient observations

A patient with heart failure may look normal when resting, or may present with an ashen complexion, and bluish or cold extremities. They are often on supplemental oxygen, and even a trip down a hall to a bathroom can cause them to pant, or break out into a sweat. They are likely to have some edema, particularly in their hands, feet, and/or lower legs.

Obviously, the goal of Asian Medicine is to start treating patients when or before they reach level I. Heart disease is one of the largest killers of adults. Ironically, it is also one of the most preventable (excluding people with congenital heart diseases). TCM emphasizes a balanced medicinal diet, and qigong exercises to maintain heart health.

"Fan hou bai bu zou, huo dao jiu shi jiu" is an ancient Chinese saying meaning, "If you take 100 steps after each meal, you'll live to be 99." Research has confirmed this practice to be beneficial, especially for patients with (non-insulin dependent) Type 2 diabetes. Although qigong is not aerobic, its series of movements help with muscle toning, balance, and blood circulation and it has an added effect of calming the mind. Practicing qigong has the added advantage of being a lifelong activity, so both the elderly and the young can enjoy this heart-healthy exercise.

Research on acupuncture and TCM for heart disease

In Traditional Chinese Medicine, angina pectoris is known as Zhen Xin Tong (true chest pain). A meta-analysis of eight clinical trials conducted between 2000 and 2014 (Zhang et al. 2016) demonstrated the efficacy of acupuncture for the treatment of stable angina (Health CMi 2016b). Electrocardiograms showed that acupuncture not only alleviated angina but it also beat the effect of cardiac drugs.

Patients in eight studies had been diagnosed with a history of stable angina pectoris for at least three months. Acupuncture treatment in all trials lasted at least one week. Some studies included additional TCM therapies such as cupping, moxibustion, and ear acupuncture. For constitutional deficiency, the acupoints UB 15 (Xinshu), UB 17 (Geshu), UB 20 (Pishu), UB 23 (Shenshu), H 7 (Shenmen), P 7 (Daling), St 36 (Zusanli), and Ren/CV 6 (Qihai) were employed. For moving stasis, the acupoints H 5 (Tongli), P 3 (Quze), P 4 (Ximen), P 5 (Jianshu), P 6 (Neiguan), and Ren/CV 17 (Danzhong) were used. Although further clinical trials are needed, there was a clear indication that acupuncture therapy may be effective and safe for treating stable angina pectoris. It was also found to be a highly effective and cost-effective adjunct therapy when used with allopathic treatments (Health CMi 2016b).

The influence of P 6 (Neiguan) on cardiovascular disorders was the subject of another study (Li *et al.* 2012). Acupuncture of P 6 (Neiguan) modulates the activity of the cardiovascular system, producing a long-lasting effect that may be attributed to the attenuation of sympathoexcitatory cardiovascular reflex responses. This explanation of the neurophysiological basis of the effects of stimulating P 6 (Neiguan) may explain its effectiveness for treating angina pectoris.

In a 2013 study, researchers found acupuncture therapy on P 6 (Neiguan) has a therapeutic effect on cardiac and chest ailments, including angina pectoris. Acupuncture points P 4 (Ximen), H 7 (Shenmen), P 7 (Daling), P 5 (Jianshi), P 3 (Quze), Ren/CV 17 (Danzhong), Ren/CV 6 (Qihai), UB 15 (Xinshu), Lu 20 (Pishu), UB 17 (Geshu), UB 23 (Shenshu), UB 16 (Ganshu), H 5 (Tongli), and St 36 (Zusanli) were found to be additionally beneficial in the treatment of angina.

Acupuncture not only quickly relieves the symptoms of acute angina pectoris, but also improves nitroglycerine's therapeutic effects. It is an efficient and simple therapeutic method which can be used for emergency (acute) and regular angina. A review of studies on acupuncture therapy has shown the effectiveness of P 6 (Neiguan) to range between 80 percent and 96.2 percent. That percentage range is almost as effective as a conventional drug regimen. It also has the obvious advantage of lacking adverse side effects commonly associated with Western antianginal drugs (Xu *et al.* 2013).

When treating a patient who has already had a heart attack, it is essential that the practitioner differentiates the pattern of disharmony. In an excellent veterinary acupuncture article, Huisheng Xie (2011) discusses how to use acupuncture for the treatment of heart failure.

The points and the formulas may be used across species. While this is not a scientific research paper, it could be used in a discussion with a Western medicine team, to illustrate how a TCM practitioner might differentiate patterns. It is a noteworthy example of the variations in clinical signs and symptoms that will determine which point prescriptions and which herbal combinations a practitioner would choose.

- For qi-blood stagnation, use points UB 14 (Jueyinshu), UB 15 (Xinshu), P 6 (Neiguan), Lu 7 (Lieque), Lu 9 (Taiyuan), H 7 (Shenmen), Liv 3 (Taichong), LI 4 (Hegu), and herbal Compound Danshen (Dripping Pills).

- If the patient has heart qi deficiency, treat with UB 14 (Jueyinshu), UB 15 (Xinshu), P 6 (Neiguan), Lu 7 (Lieque), Lu 9 (Taiyuan), H 7 (Shenmen), Ren/CV 17 (Danzhong), Ren/CV 14 (Juque), Ren/CV 4 (Guanyuan), St 36 (Zusanli), and the formula Yangxitang (Heart Qi Tonic).

- For heart yang deficiency, treat the patient with acupuncture to UB 14 (Jueyinshu), UB 15 (Xinshu), P 6 (Neiguan), Lu 7 (Lieque), Lu 9 (Taiyuan), H 7 (Shenmen), Du/GV 3 (Yaoyangguan), and Du/GV 4 (Mingmen), and moxibustion on Du/GV 20 (Baihui). For herbal treatment, use Baoyuantang (Preserve the Basal Decoction).

- In cases of kidney yang deficiency, pick UB 23 (Shenshu), UB 26 (Guanyuanshu), K 3 (Taixi), K 7 (Fuliu), Lu 7 (Lieque), Lu 9 (Taiyuan), H 7 (Shenmen), and Ren/CV 4 (Guanyuan), moxibustion on Ren/CV 6 (Qihai), plus herbal formula Zhenwutang (True Warrior Decoction).

- For deficiency of qi and yin, the author does not list points, instead he instructs practitioners to tonify heart qi and yin, activate blood, and regulate the pulse. Use the formula Shengmaiyin (Replenish Pulse Pills).

- Finally, for collapse of yang qi, use points Du/GV 26 (Shuigou), K 1 (Yongquan), SJ 5 (Waijuan), P 6 (Neiguan), LI 10 (Shousanli), and St 36 (Zusanli) with Shenfutang (Ginseng and Prepared Aconite Decoction).

In treating hospice patients, there will be times you may be limited in your choice of points due to the positioning or condition of the patient. In general, if you can only use one point on a patient with a cardiovascular disease, consider P 6 (Neiguan).

HIV/AIDS

Human immunodeficiency virus (HIV) is a virus that targets and alters the immune system, increasing the risk and impact of other infections, diseases, and some cancers. HIV is spread through contact with the blood, semen, pre-seminal fluid, rectal fluids, vaginal fluids, or breast milk of a person with HIV. Without treatment, HIV can gradually destroy the immune system and advance to AIDS (acquired immune deficiency syndrome).

Hospice criteria for HIV

For a hospice diagnosis, a patient has either 1A or 1B and 2 and 3 in the following:

1. A. CD4+ < 25 cells/μL OR

   B. Viral load > 100,000/ml

   AND

2. At least *one* of the following:

   - Central nervous system (CNS) lymphoma

   - Untreated or refractory wasting (loss of more than 33% lean body mass)

   - Mycobacterium avium complex (MAC) bacteremia

- Progressive multifocal leukoencephalopathy

- Systemic lymphoma

- Visceral kaposi sarcoma (KS)

- Renal failure, no hemodialysis (HD)

- Cryptosporidium infection

- Refractory toxoplasmosis

AND

3. PPS of < 50 percent.

More information on HIV

In the US, HIV is spread mainly by having anal or vaginal sex or sharing injection drug equipment, such as needles, with a person who has HIV. It is characterized by an extremely weakened immune system. The virus attacks and destroys the infection-fighting CD4 cells of the immune system. The loss of CD4 cells makes it difficult for the body to fight infections and certain cancers.

A person's cluster of differentiation 4 (CD4)+ T Helper cells are usually considered to be normal in a range between 500 and 1200 cells/mm^3. People with HIV, if treated, can live comfortably with 300–500 cells/mm^3. People with a CD4 count of fewer than 200 cells per microliter (μL, or equivalently, cubic millimeter, mm^3) are at high risk of contracting an AIDS-defining disease or condition. AIDS is the final stage of HIV.

A viral load is the detectable level of a virus in a quantity of blood, and is usually expressed in ml. A person can be diagnosed with HIV if their viral load is over 100,000/ml, even if their CD4+ is greater than 25 cells/μL.

Please keep in mind that as a practitioner, if you are working with a patient who is suffering from HIV, or any form of weakened immune system, you must be very strict in your use of universal precautions. A normal immune system can fight off a virus or bacteria, but you could kill someone with a compromised immune system if you exposed them to new germs.

Patient profile

Since the early 1980s, over 77.3 million individuals have been infected with HIV worldwide and an estimated 35.4 million people have died from AIDS-related illnesses (UNAIDS 2018). In the US, the majority of HIV patients are gay or bisexual men, or men who have sex with other men but do not identify themselves as gay or bisexual. African-American, Hispanic/Latino, and American Indian/Alaskan Native men are at higher risk than whites. Impoverished communities, people without health insurance, areas underserved by healthcare providers, and cultures that are unaccepting of homosexuality are at higher risk of contracting the virus. That does not mean that wealthy white heterosexual women do not get or spread the virus, only that more than half the patients diagnosed are in the previous categories.

When a patient with a weakened immune system falls prey to an opportunistic infection (OI), a doctor will diagnose the patient as having AIDS. According to a very detailed article on HIV Medical News Today (Feldman 2018), these OIs include the following:

- *Lymphoma:* Cancer of the lymph nodes and lymphoid tissues as lymphoma—there are many different types. Hodgkin and non-Hodgkin lymphoma have strong links to HIV infection.

- *Wasting syndrome:* Involuntary weight loss, including 10 percent of muscle mass, through diarrhea, weakness, or fever. Weight loss may also consist of body fat loss.

- *Mycobacteria, including mycobacterium avium and mycobacterium kansasii:* Occur naturally in the environment and pose few problems for people with fully functioning immune systems. In HIV-infected individuals (especially those with low T-cell counts), these bacteria can spread throughout the body and become life threatening.

- *Progressive multifocal leukoencephalopathy (PML):* The John Cunningham (JC) virus occurs in a vast number of people, usually lying dormant in the kidneys. In patients with compromised immune systems, either due to HIV or medications (such as those used for multiple sclerosis), the JC virus attacks the brain, leading to a dangerous condition called progressive multifocal leukoencephalopathy (PML). PML can be life threatening, causing paralysis and cognitive difficulties.

- *Kaposi's sarcoma (KS):* Kaposi's sarcoma herpesvirus (KSHV), also known as human herpesvirus 8 (HHV-8), causes a cancer that leads to the growth of abnormal blood vessels anywhere in the body. KS appears as solid purple or pink spots on the surface of the skin. They can be flat or raised. Lesions may appear internally in the digestive system or lungs. New anti-viral and cancer drugs are making KS less life threatening.

- *Cryptosporidiosis:* The protozoan parasite Cryptosporidium causes an infection that leads to severe abdominal cramps and watery diarrhea.

- *Toxoplasmosis (toxo):* Toxoplasma gondii is a parasite that inhabits warm-blooded animals, including cats and rodents, and leaves the body in their feces. Humans contract the diseases by inhaling contaminated dust or eating contaminated food (it can occur in commercial meats). T. gondii causes severe infection in the lungs, retina, heart, liver, pancreas, brain, testes, and colon. Wearing protective gloves and a mask when changing cat litter and thoroughly washing the hands afterward can stop exposure, but for immunocompromised individuals, it is best to avoid exposure.

Other serious infections and diseases that lead to a diagnosis of AIDS include:

- *Candidiasis of the bronchi, trachea, esophagus, and lungs:* As a fungal infection that normally occurs in the skin and nails, this frequently causes serious problems in the esophagus and lower respiratory tract for people with AIDS.

- *Invasive cervical cancer:* This type of cancer begins in the cervix and metastasizes to other areas in the body; it can spread faster in immunosuppressed patients, but is normally found in routine check-ups.

- *Coccidioidomycosis:* People sometimes refer to the self-limited version of this disease in healthy individuals as valley fever. Inhalation of the fungus Coccidioides immitis causes this infection.

- *Cryptococcosis:* Cryptococcus neoformans is a fungus that can infect any part of the body, but most often enters the lungs to trigger pneumonia. It can also enter the brain, causing encephalopathy.

- *Cytomegalovirus disease (CMV):* This can cause a range of diseases in the body, including pneumonia, gastroenteritis, and encephalitis, a brain infection. CMV retinitis is of particular concern in people with late-stage HIV, as it infects the retina at the back of the eye, permanently removing sight. CMV retinitis is a medical emergency.

- *HIV-related encephalopathy:* An acute or chronic HIV infection can trigger this brain disorder. While doctors do not fully understand the cause, they consider it to be linked to post-infection inflammation in the brain.

- *Herpes simplex (HSV):* This virus, usually sexually transmitted or passed on in childbirth, is extremely common and rarely causes health issues in people with healthy immune systems. It can reactivate in people with HIV, causing painful cold sores around the mouth and ulcers on the genitals and anus that do not resolve. The sores are an indicator that HIV has become AIDS. HSV may also infect the breathing tube, lungs, or esophagus of people with AIDS.

- *Histoplasmosis:* The fungus Histoplasma capsulatum causes extremely severe, pneumonia-like symptoms in people with advanced HIV. This condition can become progressive disseminated histoplasmosis, which includes generalized involvement of the reticuloendothelial system, with hepato-splenomegaly, lymphadenopathy, bone marrow involvement, and sometimes oral or gastrointestinal ulcerations. In HIV patients, the central nervous system may become involved, causing meningitis or focal brain lesions.

- *Chronic intestinal isosporiasis:* The parasite Isospora belli can infect the body through contaminated food and water, causing diarrhea, fever, vomiting, weight loss, headaches, and abdominal pain.

- *Tuberculosis (TB):* The bacteria Mycobacterium tuberculosis causes this disease and can transfer in droplets if a person with an active form of the bacteria sneezes, coughs, or speaks. TB causes a severe lung infection as well as weight loss, fever, and tiredness, and can also infect the brain, lymph nodes, bones, or kidneys.

- *Pneumocystis jirovecii pneumonia (PJP):* A fungus called Pneumocystis jirovecii causes breathlessness, dry cough, and high fever in people with suppressed immune systems, including those with HIV.

- *Recurrent pneumonia:* Many different infections can cause pneumonia, but a bacteria called Streptococcus pneumoniae is one of its most dangerous causes in people with HIV. Vaccines are available for this bacterium, and every person who has HIV should receive vaccination for Streptococcus pneumoniae.

- *Recurrent Salmonella septicemia:* This type of bacteria often enters the body in contaminated food and water, circulates the entire body, and overpowers the immune system, causing nausea, diarrhea, and vomiting.

Antiretroviral drugs (ARVs)

Felman (2018) goes on to discuss the treatment of HIV involving antiretroviral medications that fight the HIV infection and slows down the spread of the virus in the body. People living with HIV generally take a combination of medications called highly active antiretroviral therapy (HAART) or combination antiretroviral therapy (cART).

There are a number of subgroups of antiretrovirals, such as:

- *Protease inhibitors:* Protease is an enzyme that HIV needs to replicate. These medications bind to the enzyme and inhibit its action, preventing HIV from making copies of itself. These include:

  - Atazanavir/Cobicistat (Evotaz)

  - Lopinavir/Ritonavir (Kaletra)

  - Darunavir/Cobicistat (Prezcobix).

- *Integrase inhibitors:* HIV needs integrase, another enzyme, to infect T-cells. These drugs block integrase. These are often the first line of treatment due to their effectiveness and limited side effects for many people. Integrase inhibitors include:

  - Elvitegravir (Vitekta)

  - Dolutegravir (Tivicay)

  - Raltegravir (Isentress).

- *Nucleoside/nucleotide reverse transcriptase inhibitors (NRTIs):* These drugs, also referred to as "nukes," interfere with HIV as it tries to replicate. This class of drugs includes:

  - Abacavir (Ziagen)

  - Lamivudine/Zidovudine (Combivir)

  - Emtricitabine (Emtriva)

  - Tenofovir disproxil (Viread).

- *Non-nucleoside reverse transcriptase inhibitors (NNRTIs):* These work in a similar way to NRTIs, making it more difficult for HIV to replicate.

- *Chemokine co-receptor antagonists:* These drugs block HIV from entering cells. However, doctors in the US do not often prescribe these because other drugs are more effective.

- *Entry inhibitors:* Entry inhibitors prevent HIV from entering T-cells. Without access to these cells, HIV cannot replicate. As with chemokine co-receptor antagonists, they are not common in the US.

People will often use a combination of these drugs to suppress HIV. A medical team will adapt the exact mix of drugs to each individual. Those mixes are commonly known as "cocktails." HIV treatment is usually permanent, lifelong, and based on routine dosage. A person living with HIV must take pills on a regular schedule. Each class of antiretroviral drugs has different side effects, but possible common side effects include:

- Nausea

- Fatigue

- Diarrhea

- Headache

- Skin rashes.

Complementary or alternative medicine

Felman (2018) boldly claimed, "Although many people who have HIV try complementary, alternative, or herbal options, such as herbal remedies, no evidence confirms them to be effective." However, that conclusion is in direct contradiction to much of the research on HIV and AIDS. He goes on to say, "According to some limited studies, mineral or vitamin supplements may provide some benefits in overall health. It is important to discuss these options with a healthcare provider because some of these options, even vitamin supplements, may interact with ARVs." That statement does appear to be true, and any herbs prescribed for HIV patients should be checked against their current prescriptions.

Acupuncture and TCM research on HIV

In China, it is standard practice for HIV patients to use TCM treatments. When polled, patients cited the following reasons for using TCM: having an expectation of a good effect, reduction of symptoms from the disease or from the side effect of the medications, a desire for improvement in quality of life, and control over the disease process. Evidence from experimental studies and clinical trials has demonstrated a positive association between the use of TCM and immune promotion or symptom relief of people living with HIV/AIDS.

TCM puts stress on the reactivity and adaptability of the body to pathogens. In TCM, patients are treated with different therapies, including Chinese drugs, acupuncture, moxibustion, and qigong exercise. These treatments aim to elevate the quality of life and prolong the lifespan of patients. Therapies enhance the immune function of the organism, block the development of the virus, and retard the initiation (the progression from the asymptomatic stage to the AIDS stage). Additionally, they can alleviate the symptoms and signs of the disease.

Peripheral neuropathy is one of the most common neurological complications of HIV infection, and diarrhea is another common symptom (Anastasi *et al.* 2011). According to a British Acupuncture Factsheet on Acupuncture and HIV Infection (British Acupuncture Council 2012), acupuncture acts on areas of the brain known to reduce sensitivity to pain and stress. It works by deactivating the "analytical" brain, responsible for anxiety and worry, by increasing the release of adenosine. For the treatment of peripheral neuropathy, it increases local microcirculation, which aids in the dispersal of swelling. By releasing vascular and immunomodulatory factors, it reduces inflammation.

In an unrelated study (Shiflett and Schwartz 2011), acupuncture was associated with reduced attrition and mortality rates in patients suffering from HIV infection.

Two randomized controlled trials (Chang and Sommers 2011; Chang *et al.* 2007) found that there could potentially be synergistic effects of acupuncture and relaxation, one for treating gastrointestinal symptoms and the other to improve quality of life. In other acupuncture research, treatments were credited with a positive effect on other neuropathic pain. Further clinical trials are needed, but acupuncture has been reported by HIV patients to help facial pain, diarrhea, and sleep disturbance. The addition of moxibustion appeared to increase total lymphocyte count (British Acupuncture Council 2012).

Gastrointestinal symptoms are often the major side effect of medications for HIV. Boosting the immune system is not the only benefit of Asian Medicine. Increasing patient compliance always results in better outcomes.

Acupuncture eases side effects of AIDS drugs

In 2005, a study (Laino 2005) presented at a meeting of the International AIDS Society included 50 HIV-infected men and women taking HIV medications. About half had been diagnosed with full-blown AIDS. Of those 50 patients, nearly 80 percent had gas, more than 40 percent had bloating, 50 percent had cramps, nearly 50 percent had appetite loss, and 10 percent had actually lost weight.

Participants received six weeks of acupuncture. For three weeks, the acupuncture included four sites commonly associated with improvement of digestive symptoms such as nausea, vomiting, and bowel upset; for another three weeks, they received acupuncture at four nearby sites not noted for affecting digestive conditions.

Both sets of acupuncture points improved digestive symptoms. However, acupuncture at the sites targeting digestive symptoms was more effective in controlling loss of appetite, abdominal cramps, and bloating. This is an essential finding, because the number one reason patients are non-compliant with their AIDS medications is the gastrointestinal side effects of the drugs. Although this study did not mention which points were used, it did show symptom improvements with the use of acupuncture. In addition, three RCT trials reported that warming moxibustion to the main points—Ren/CV 8 (Sheque), Ren/CV 4 (Guanyuan), St 36 (Zusanli), Ren/CV

12 (Zhongwan), and St 25 (Tianshu)—produced positive effects on AIDS patients with diarrhea.

Miriam Lee (1992) has a 12-day moxibustion treatment that begins with similar points in Appendix E of her book *Insights of a Senior Acupuncturist*. It should be noted that she cautions against needling, not for fear of contamination, but because any form of needling can cause drainage, and the patient with AIDS is already in a very depleted state. The same warning should be heeded for any frail patient, and moxibustion or other warming techniques may be the better treatment choice.

Another physician, Hal Huff, ND, a naturopathic doctor at the Canadian College of Naturopathic Medicine in Toronto, says: "We give acupuncture in conjunction with other treatments such as dietary changes and nutritional supplements, so I can't say for certain whether it's acupuncture or the whole package that results in improvement, but people report fewer digestive problems and improved compliance with their AIDS medications."

TCM has something to offer HIV patients with herbal medicine as well. Three double-blind RCTs (Wang and Zou 2010) reported that HIV RNA levels were significantly reduced after six months to one year of regular doses of Chinese herbs (Compound SH, Tangcao Tablets, Qiankunning Capsule). Tangcao tablets were the first patent formulas approved by the State Food and Drug Administration (SFDA) for alleviating the symptoms and signs of HIV/AIDS patients. At the time that report was written, five other relatively matured compounds were still under trial.

Given the body of evidence above, it is safe to conclude that TCM appears to be associated with the improvement in immune function and quality of life, and some symptom control for AIDS-related opportunistic diseases, as well as offering relief for some medication-related side effects.

Liver disease

End-stage liver disease includes a subgroup of patients with cirrhosis (scarring of the liver—hard scar tissue replaces soft healthy tissue) who have signs of decompensation that is generally irreversible with medical management other than transplant. Decompensation includes hepatic encephalopathy, variceal bleed, kidney impairment, ascites, and lung issues.

Hospice criteria for liver disease

Patients will be considered to be in the terminal stage of liver disease if they meet the following criteria: 1 and 2 must be present; factors from 3 will lend supporting documentation.

1. The patient has end-stage liver disease as evidenced by the following:

   - Prothrombin time prolonged more than five seconds over control

   or both of the following:

   - International Normalized Ratio (INR) > 1.5

   - Serum albumin < 2.5gm/dl.

2. The patient shows at least *one* of the following:

   - Ascites, refractory to treatment or patient non-compliant

   - Spontaneous bacterial peritonitis

   - Hepatorenal syndrome (elevated creatinine and blood urea nitrogen (BUN) with oliguria (< 400ml/day) and urine sodium concentration)

   - Hepatic encephalopathy, refractory to treatment or patient non-compliant

   - Recurrent variceal bleeding, despite intensive therapy.

3. Documentation of the following factors will support eligibility for hospice care:

   - Progressive malnutrition

   - Muscle wasting with reduced strength and endurance

- Continued active alcoholism (> 80gm ethanol/day)

- Hepatocellular carcinoma

- HBsAg (hepatitis B) positivity

- Hepatitis C, refractory to interferon treatment.

More information on liver disease

Much like heart disease, some causative factors of liver disease can be avoided with prevention and treatment. For instance, alcohol-induced cirrhosis, viral hepatitis, obesity, and drugs that are known to damage the liver are now generally avoidable. End-stage liver disease may also be caused by non-alcoholic cirrhosis, genetic disorders, cancer of the liver, and autoimmune disorders, which are less controllable and are therefore non-preventable factors.

A liver transplant is the only chance most people have to survive end-stage liver disease. The decompensated liver disease allows these patients to be prioritized on the transplant list. Patients awaiting liver transplant who otherwise fit the above criteria may be certified for the Medicare hospice benefit, but if a donor organ is procured, the patient must be discharged from the hospice.

Like most cancers, the beginning stages of liver disease can be painless, and symptom free. Even if the liver becomes inflamed while fighting a virus, it might not be painful. In turn, if that inflammation leads to fibrosis, the symptoms may also go unnoticed. Often, a patient reaches the level of having some cirrhosis before outward clinical signs appear. A blockage may occur, causing blood to back up in the vessels supplying the liver. Left unnoticed or untreated, these blood vessels may burst. The patient may bruise easily, or bleed freely. Other clinically significant signs can include edema in the legs, ascites in the abdomen, jaundice leading to a yellow discoloration in the skin and the sclera of eyes, and intense itching of the skin (Seladi-Schulman 2019).

Decreased inability to filter the blood can lead to an increased half-life of medications. This variance in the normal absorption and other irregularities in the distribution of medications can lead to increased sensitivity to medications and a worsening of side effects.

Both the kidneys and the liver filter toxins from the blood. Diseases of the liver can lead to insulin-resistance, which leads to Type 2 diabetes. Furthermore, if left untreated, toxins can accumulate in the brain. Rising ammonia levels result in problems with concentration, memory, sleeping, or other mental functions. Patients are often prescribed lactulose to move the bowels in an attempt to lower their ammonia levels.

Patient profiles

Patient A is a 78-year-old male. He has a known history of 60+ years of alcoholism and tobacco dependency. He had a recent rupture of esophageal varices that resulted in a hospital stay of several days, requiring transfusions. He has been ordered by his physician to stop smoking and limit his alcohol consumption to one can of beer a day. Currently he is on 2 liters of oxygen, but does not always use it when he goes out for walks, and is often non-compliant with the one beer per day limit. He has a strong family and veterans support group. He is not eligible for a liver transplant.

Patient B is a 50-year-old female who has no history of alcohol or tobacco use. She has a 23-year history of hepatitis B from a blood transfusion she received after the birth of her third child. She has always maintained a healthy diet, and utilized Asian Medicine to maintain a balance system. She was diagnosed five years ago after experiencing overwhelming fatigue. Patient B has the very strong support of family and friends. She is not expected to survive unless she receives a liver transplant, for which she is eligible.

They are both placed in hospice care.

Patient A is in the hospice for six weeks. There is questionable compliance with his limit on alcohol consumption, and he admits to smoking occasionally. He is hopeful, and makes plans to visit his sister in three weeks, where he is looking forward to "laying back on a raft in the pool and taking a nap floating in the sunshine."

Patient A takes an unannounced trip out of town, with a known "drinking buddy." He falls into an old pattern, and participates in three days of binge-drinking and chain-smoking. Two days after he returns home, he has had several cans of beer and begins to have violent abdominal cramping, followed by bloody diarrhea; after 30 minutes, he calls his daughter. The daughter arrives 20 minutes later and she calls the hospice nurse, to report he is vomiting what looks like bile, feces, and blood. He has collapsed on the floor, and is too weak to answer her, or stand up.

The nurse arrives 15 minutes later to find him unresponsive; his eyes are extremely jaundiced and he is actively dying from internal hemorrhaging. After her examination, she calls the medical director who confirms that the patient has most likely suffered completed and irreversible liver failure. He slips into a coma and dies 45 minutes after the nurse arrives, from what she describes as one of the "worst deaths she has ever witnessed."

Patient B is in the hospice two weeks before she finds out she is lucky enough to picked for a new drug trial (this case was prior to the latest hepatitis B medication). The medication is extremely expensive, but it cures her of hepatitis. The side effects leave her with non-alcoholic liver cirrhosis and extreme joint damage. Her liver enzyme results are very bad and she is warned that she could still die waiting for a transplant.

She is an acupuncturist and herbalist who works with Chinese herbs and mushrooms to tonify and balance her liver qi. On a follow-up visit to her doctor, staff are amazed because her laboratory results for her liver enzymes have come back into the normal range. She is told this never happens with people who have had cirrhosis. This recovery takes place over a year. She is taken off the transplant list, and discharged from hospice care.

Acupuncture and Chinese herbal medicine for liver disease

Acupuncture and herbs are used preventatively to treat liver functions before a patient reaches the stages of chronic or acute liver diseases, but what about more advanced cases?

In one study (Health CMi 2016a), researchers from Nanyang City First People's Hospital (Henan Province, China) tested a TCM protocol using acupuncture, far infrared heat therapy, herbal intravenous injections, herbal soba noodle soup, and a herbal oral decoction for the treatment of end-stage liver cirrhosis and ascites. The treatment protocol reduced or eliminated ascites, improved urine volume and appetite, and normalized liver and kidney function, proving acupuncture and herbs are effective for the treatment of cirrhosis with ascites.

In the protocol, patients received acupuncture once a day for 30 days. The points needled were Sp 9 (Yinlingquan), Sp 6 (Sanyinjiao), K 3 (Taixi), Liv 3 (Taichong), and Ren/CV 4 (Guanyuan). After de qi was achieved, mild reinforcing and reducing techniques were utilized. To maintain de qi, the needles were manually stimulated every ten minutes. Each acupuncture session lasted 30 minutes.

During the daily acupuncture session, a TDP (Te-Ding Dian-ci-bo Pu, Chinese for "Special Electromagnetic Spectrum") heat lamp (far infrared with a special mineralized plate) was focused on Ren/CV 4 (Guanyuan). In addition, the point was manually stimulated using a tonification technique to bring de qi to the point.

The patients received IV fluids consisting of 40ml of Hong Hua extract and 250ml of 5 percent glucose once every day for one month.

In addition, a herbal decoction was administered once a day for one month. The amount of the herbs was not disclosed, but the crude herbs consisted of:

Qing Hao (Herba Artemisiae Annuae)

Tong Cao (Medulla Tetrapanacis Papyriferi)

Dan Shen (Radix Salviae Miltiorrhizae)

Wang Bu Liu Xing (Semen Vaccariae Segetalis)

Hou Po (Cortex Magnoliae Officinalis)

Si Gua Luo (Fasciculus Vascularis Luffae)

Sheng Di Huang (Radix Rehmanniae Glutinosae)

Shi Hu (Herba Dendrobii)

Che Qian Zi (Semen Plantaginis)

Dang Gui (Radix Angelicae Sinensis)

Bai Zhu (Rhizoma Atractylodis Macrocephalae)

Yu Jin (Tuber Curcumae)

Da Fu Pi (Pericarpium Arecae Catechu)

Lian Qiao (Fructus Forsythiae Suspensae)

Di Long (Lumbricus)

Chen Xiang (Lignum Aquilariae).

It should be noted here that some of the herbs in the decoction have very strong purging properties and may not be suitable for patients in weakened conditions.

Finally, a soup consisting of herbs and soba noodles was consumed once a day for three days. The recipe called for the herbs to be baked and ground into a powder by using equal parts (75g) of:

Gan Sui (Radix Euphorbiae Kansui)

Hong Da Ji, Da Ji (Radix Euphorbiae seu Knoxiae)

Yuan Hua (Flos Daphnes Genkwa)

Qian Nui Zi (Semen Pharbitidis).

To make the combination, 10g of the baked, ground herb mix was added to 60g of soba noodle flour to create the noodles. The noodles were then added to boiling water and the broth and noodles were consumed.

The conclusion of the 30-day study showed that acupuncture and herbs were effective for the treatment of liver cirrhosis and hepatosplenomegaly (enlargement of the liver and spleen).

Furthermore, acupuncture with moxibustion is effective for the treatment of cirrhosis with ascites.

In another study (Price 2011), entitled "Enhancing xenobiotic detox," acupuncture performed well as an acupuncture-herb combination in reducing the clinical symptoms of liver cirrhosis. A xenobiotic is a chemical substance found within an organism that is not naturally produced or expected to be there (in this case they were referring to ammonia). In this study, the acupuncture and herb combination did better than treatments with glucuronolactone (a drug often used for detoxification purposes) or glucuronolactone-lamivudine (a nucleoside analogue reverse transcriptase inhibitor).

Unfortunately, they did not mention the herbs used. The acupuncture points applied were UB 18 (Ganshu), the liver back-shu point near the T9 spine ganglion that corresponds to part of the liver innervation; LI 14 (Binao), the front-mu point of the liver; K 3 (Taixi) which tonifies liver yin; and Sp 6 (Sanyinjiao), the crossing point of the spleen, kidney, and liver meridians.

Do these points sound familiar? They are all Hospice Acupuncture Protocol points.

It was previously noted that toxins in the blood can affect the brain, but what happens when the medications or other treatments become minimally effective? Hepatic encephalopathy (HE) is defined as a spectrum of neuropsychiatric abnormalities in patients with liver dysfunction. The primary cause of HE is believed to be an increase in harmful substances, ammonia, γ-aminobutyric acid (GABA), false neurotransmitters entering the brain via the blood, and the imbalance of certain amino acids in plasma. It is diagnosed after excluding other forms of brain disease. Hepatic encephalopathy is characterized by personality changes, intellectual impairment, and a depressed level of consciousness. The aggravation of HE will result in coma hepaticum, commonly known as a hepatic coma, which may ultimately lead to death.

In an article on evidence-based complementary and alternative medicine, Chun Yao and colleagues (2012) shared the following insights on management of HE with Traditional Chinese Medicine. TCM defines HE as invasion of damp heat in the triple burners leading to phlegm, and qi stagnation that eventually clouds the ability to think clearly in HE patients. Although one should be discouraged from generalizing, HE patients usually have advanced chronic liver disease and it is safe to assume that they will present with many of the physical and laboratory stigmata associated with severe hepatic dysfunction. General signs and symptoms include muscle wasting, jaundice, ascites, palmar erythema, spider telangiectasias (dilated small blood vessels in the skin or mucous membranes, also called spider veins), and fetor (or feoeter) hepaticus. Fetor hepaticus is also called the "breath of death," and is described as a musty, sweet breath which some liken to a combination of garlic and rotten eggs.

It is essential to examine the patient and assess for various patterns of disharmony to determine your treatment. General nutritional considerations for all patterns should include restricting protein intake, maintaining hydration, and reducing the pH of the blood by adding vitamin C to help divert ammonia away from the brain and into the bloodstream. TCM includes purgation and eliminating stasis in organs and inducing resuscitation, which is holistic and dynamic in nature.

Chun Yao *et al.* made the following HE-related patterns and herbal recommendations for treatment:

> Invasion of the pericardium by excessive heat toxin—Purple Snowy Powder, Qing Yig Liang Xue Tang and Cow-bezoar Bolus for Resurrection, Anti Pyretic and Antitoxic Decoction, Coptidis Decoction for Detoxification, combined with Rhubarb and Treasured Bolus.

> Dampness and Phlegm Accumulation Causing Mental Confusion—Herbae Artemisiae Capillariae Decoction, Artemisiae Scopariae and Poriae Powder, Phlegm-removing decoction, combined with Rhubarb and Storax Pill, Jufang Zhibao Dan, Yin Chen Si Ling Decoction and Changpu Yijin Decoction.

> Yin deficiency of liver and kidney coupled with yang excess of liver—Du Xiao Ke Li, Yiguan Decoction, Cornu Satgae and Subphrenic Recesses.

> Exhaustion of yin and yang coupled with Disturbance in Spirit—Pulse-Activating Powder or Cornus Rhinoceri and Rehmanniae Decoction, Shen Fu Long Mu Tang, or Ginseng Decoction. (Yao *et al.* 2012, pp.4–5)

Section 4.2 of the paper, entitled "Purging organs and opening orifices," offers an excellent summation of HE, and offers a potent herbal solution:

The pathogenesis of HE mostly includes the deficiency of liver and kidney, phlegm retention and blood stasis, failure of Yang and Yin to raise and fall, respectively, which could be regarded as the declining function in distributing nutrients to the organ and excretion out of the organ, leading to the symptoms like coma, convulsion, and mental confusion.

The main cause of liver failure is a combination of toxin, phlegm, and blood stasis entangled in the body along with dampness, and pestilence invasion. Removing toxins, expelling blood stasis, and eliminating phlegm have been applied in clinical treatment of HE.

Rhubarb (Rhei Radix and Rhizoma) is a potent herb with purging activity, which can relieve internal heat and promote blood circulation by removing blood stasis and normalizing gallbladder to cure jaundice.

30g of Rhubarb was prepared to decoction in 200ml of water as an enema. 1–2 times daily for 10 days as a course of treatment. "Complete remedy" (CR) was defined as reaching and maintaining a conscious and lucid state of mind for 3 weeks after dose.

One study was conducted with a group of 64 patients with HE, in an attempt to relieve internal heat, and cool, promote blood flow, eliminate phlegm, and free channels. Patients were divided into two equal groups. The control group subjects received intravenous infusion of 40ml of Qingkailing (a TCM drug) injection, 250ml of BCAA or 10g of Hepa Merz, once a day. The second group, the TCM patients, received Tongfu Xiere Decoction in addition to the treatments in the control group. The decoction was prepared as an enema and administered through colon infusion at 250ml a day. Tongfu Xiere Decoction contains Rhubarb, Dandelion, Magnolia Bark, Citri Immaturus, and Fructus Mume.

The therapeutic efficacy in the TCM group reached 93.94 percent, while the control group reached 80.65 percent. (Yao *et al.* 2012)

No universally effective treatment has been generated in modern medicine. However, the successful use of TCM therapeutic approaches over the past decades suggests that alternative approaches should be taken into consideration for HE therapy. The treatments can be multi-leveled, employing holistic and personalized pathways in an adjustable strategy.

Acupuncture can be helpful for mild to moderate hepatitis. In a two-week study of 60 hospitalized patients with mild to moderate hepatitis B, half of the patients received daily 30-minute electroacupuncture treatments tailored to their specific TCM pattern of disharmony. The other 30 received regular Western medical treatment. The TCM group had greater rates of improvement, as evidenced by significantly shorter time for recovery of the hepatic functions, and the IL-8 level was significantly lower in patients who received EA. IL-8 is the abbreviation for interleukin 8, which has been used as a marker of liver diagnosis in various types of hepatitis.

This review has provided some insight into the formulation of points for acupuncture supplementations of liver detoxification. Practitioners must choose a combination appropriate to the pattern of disharmony, after a thorough assessment. That being said, the following points seem to be useful for targeting the liver and soothing inflammation: Liv 3 (Taichong), Liv 8 (Ququan), Liv 14 (Qimen), GB 26 (Daimai), GB 34 (Yanglingquan), St 25 (Tianshu), St 36 (Zusanli), St 40 (Fenglong), LI 4 (Hegu), P 6 (Neiguan), UB 18 (Ganshu), Ren/CV 12 (Zhongwan), and the Gan auricular point. The great auricular nerve (GAN) provides sensory innervation to the skin around the auricle.

One cautionary reminder regarding liver disease is that hepatitis is a particularly strong virus that can live outside the body on moist surfaces for prolonged periods. There are multiple strains of hepatitis, and it has proven to be quite adaptable, mutational, and difficult to destroy. A common practice in treating patients with addictions is to employ the National Acupuncture Detoxification Association (NADA) Protocol using auricular acupuncture. In this form of treatment, the patients use a mirror to remove their own needles and place them in a safe waste container, and there is a supply of clean cotton balls they can apply to their ears if they have any bleeding. This greatly decreases the risk of any accidental needle sticks, and cross-contamination.

As a note on prevention, acupuncture can help with active alcoholism and drug addiction. NADA has years of scientific and experiential evidence showing that auricular acupuncture can help patients actively detoxify from drugs and alcohol by treating the patient's signs and symptoms of withdrawal. Patients who undergo ongoing auricular acupuncture are more likely to complete a drug treatment program, and less likely to relapse.

An imbalance in the brain's chemistry which leads to a deficiency of neurotransmitters is the cause of most forms of chemical addiction. The use of intravenous amino acids has shown promising results in the treatment of alcoholics. When the brain chemistry is balanced, a person does not crave drugs or alcohol. It is a physiological condition, often genetic in origin, that manifests in addictive behaviors proven to be detrimental to a person's mental, physical, and social well-being. It is also a major cause of liver disease.

In summation, it is important to remember that all substances that enter the body are filtered by the kidneys or the liver. Acupuncture and Chinese herb therapies can be prescribed for the prevention of liver disharmonies, and to bring the body back to balance. Equally important, one must realize that a compromised liver may not be able to metabolize medications. When liver disease is advanced enough to cloud thinking, acupuncture and purgative herbs have proven to be effective for reducing edema and ascites, and restoring mental clarity.

Neurological disease

Neurological disorders are diseases of the brain, spine, and the nerves that connect them. There are more than 600 diseases of the nervous system, such as brain tumors, epilepsy, Parkinson's disease, and stroke, as well as less familiar ones such as frontotemporal dementia.

Hospice criteria for neurological diseases

Criteria are very similar for chronic degenerative conditions such as amyotrophic lateral sclerosis (ALS, also known as motor neurone disease), muscular dystrophy, multiple sclerosis, or myasthenia gravitas. Patients will be considered to be in the terminal stage of ALS if they meet the following criteria (must fulfill 1, 2, or 3):

1. The patient must demonstrate critically impaired breathing capacity with *all* of the following characteristics in the past 12 months preceding initial hospice certification:

   - Vital capacity (VC) < 30 percent of normal

   - Significant dyspnea at rest

   - Requiring supplemental oxygen even when resting (sitting or in bed)

   - Patient declines artificial ventilation

   OR

2. The patient must demonstrate both:

   a. Rapid progression of ALS as demonstrated by all of the following within the 12 months preceding initial hospice certification:

      - Progression from independent ambulation to wheelchair or bedbound status

      - Progression from normal to barely intelligible or unintelligible speech

      - Progression from normal to pureed diet

      - Progression from independence in most or all activities of daily living (ADLs) to needing major assistance by caretaker in all ADLs.

   b. Critical nutritional impairment as demonstrated by *all* of the following within the 12 months preceding initial hospice certification:

- Oral intake of nutrients and fluids insufficient to sustain life

- Continuing weight loss

- Dehydration or hypovolemia

- Absence of artificial feeding methods

OR

3. Both of the following:

   a. Rapid progression of ALS (2a above).

   b. Life-threatening complications as demonstrated by one of the following within the last 12 months preceding initial hospice certification:

      - Recurrent aspiration pneumonia (with or without tube feedings)

      - Upper UTI, e.g. pyelonephritis

      - Sepsis

      - Recurrent fever after antibiotic therapy

      - Decubitus ulcers, multiple, Stage 3–4.

More information on neurological diseases

Amyotrophic lateral sclerosis is also known as Lou Gehrig's disease, named after the famous New York Yankees baseball player who played from 1923 to 1939 and died from ALS at the age of 37. ALS is a rare, fatal, progressive degenerative disease that affects pyramidal motor neurons. It usually begins in middle age, and is characterized especially by increasing and spreading muscular weakness. In end-stage ALS, two factors are critical in determining prognosis: ability to breathe and, to a lesser extent, ability to swallow (Dharmananda 1999).

Muscular dystrophy is not one disease, but a group of over 30 genetic-based muscle diseases which have in common the weakening of muscles. The severity of the weakness varies in onset speed and muscles affected. As the disease progresses, the patient may lose the ability to walk or to breathe without assistance. Further progression of muscular dystrophy can affect the heart muscles, causing the patient to die.

Multiple sclerosis (MS) is a demyelinating disease that affects the myelin sheath of the neurons in the brain and spinal cord. It can also cause the destruction of the immune system. This progression in turn leads to motor and visual problems, as well as mental and psychiatric changes. The patient may have periods of remission, where they are symptom free from muscle weakness and decreased sensation and coordination. There are two major types of MS, one that is progressive and one that is recurrent.

Myasthenia gravis is caused by a breakdown in the normal communication between nerves and muscles. The immune system produces antibodies that block or destroy many of the muscles' receptor sites for acetylcholine. Damaged receptors lead to fewer signals being received, and, in turn, weaker muscles. Symptoms include generalized muscular weakness and rapid fatigue of voluntary muscles. Myasthenia gravis is known to start on the head, affecting the eyes and causing a facial droop.

Parkinson's disease is a disorder of the central nervous system that affects motor movement, often including tremors. Generally, decline in a patient with Parkinson's disease will manifest as difficulty with swallowing, which can lead to aspiration, and/or pneumonia, which in turn may lead to death. There is a saying in the Parkinson's disease community: "You die with Parkinson's, not from it."

Patient profile

Like all the other diseases we have discussed, there is no typical patient. The patient with ALS will not present the same way as a patient with Parkinson's. However, there are some factors about ALS patients we can generalize. They usually are diagnosed between the ages of 40 and 70, with the average age around 55. Twenty percent more men than women get ALS, and 93 percent of the people who are in the national database are Caucasian. Also, people who have served in the military are more likely than civilians to be diagnosed, especially Gulf War veterans. The cost and level of care for ALS patients can be very high, because as the disease progresses, they have less ability to carry out the activities of daily living and often become bedbound quickly. The majority of people with ALS die within two to five years of diagnosis of the disease. The exceptions to this statistic are the 10 percent of ALS patients who live 10 years or more, and the 5 percent of patients who live 20 years or longer (Dharmananda 1999).

Acupuncture research on neurological diseases

Neuropathic pain is present in many forms of disease. Although not linked to specific neurological diseases, the following findings on generalized neuropathic pain are noteworthy and may be useful in other clinical treatments:

- One systematic review of randomized controlled trials comparing acupuncture with carbamazepine for trigeminal neuralgia found acupuncture to be as effective as the drug treatment.

- Electroacupuncture was found not to be effective for chronic painful neuropathy in general.

- Acupuncture was found to be more effective than cobamamide for peripheral neuropathy due to chemotherapy.

- Acupuncture plus acupoint injection was found to be more effective than carbamazepine for greater occipital neuralgia.

- Other non-randomized studies have found encouraging results with acupuncture for chemotherapy-induced neuropathy, HIV/AIDS-induced neuropathy, trigeminal neuralgia, and peripheral neuropathy of undefined etiology.

In general, acupuncture is believed to stimulate the nervous system and cause the release of neurochemical messenger molecules. These chemicals influence the body's homeostatic mechanisms, thus promoting physical and emotional well-being (British Acupuncture Council 2014).

Treating ALS with an acupuncture approach is, as with most debilitating disease, best tried when the patient is in the earliest stages of the disease. The following paragraphs are highlights from a study (Sudhakaran 2017) with a 55-year-old woman who had weakness in her right arm and both legs for four months when she began treatment. Normally, one study with one person would not be worth mentioning, but the information and treatment strategy led the researcher to believe that "acupuncture can be an effective modality of treatment for ALS, producing symptomatic relief and improving quality of life" (p.265). Furthermore, the point selections could be clinically relevant for formulating a treatment protocol.

ALS is the most common motor neuron disease (MND). The term MND is more widely used in Europe. The presentations are:

- *ALS:* (most common) with the loss of upper motor neurons (UMN) and lower motor neurons (LMN), producing a mixed picture in the limbs. ALS can also present with a *bulbar onset*, manifesting in speech and swallowing difficulties, and limb manifestations later.

- *Progressive muscular atrophy (PMA):* predominantly with LMN lesions.

- *Primary lateral sclerosis (PLS):* predominantly with UMN lesions; this is rare.

Commonly used points to address ALS include:

- For the upper extremity: LI 15 (Jianyu), LI 14 (Binao), LI 11 (Quchi), LI 10 (Shousanli), SJ 5 (Weiguan), LI 4 (Hegu), and SI 3 are used according to the areas involved.

- For the lower extremity: GB 30 (Huantiao), GB 31 (Fengshi), St 31 (Biguan), St 32 (Futu), St 36 (Zusanli), St 41 (Jiexi), GB 41 (Zulinqi), and GB 40 (Qiuxu) are used according to location.

- GB 34 (Yanglingquan) is used in all cases of atrophy syndrome, as this is the influential point for muscles and tendons in general.

- St 30 (Qichong) tonifies the stomach channel and promotes the flow of qi to all limbs.

- UB 32 (Ciliao) and Du/GV 3 (Yaoyangguan) stimulate circulation of qi in the legs.

- Du/GV channel points: The main points used are Du/GV 16 where the Du/GV channel enters the brain, and Du/GV 20 (Baihui), Du/GV 1 (Changqiang), Du/GV 3 (Yaoyangguan), Du/GV 14 (Dazhui), and Du/GV 12 (Shenzhu).

Dermatome charts may be utilized to reference the relationship of the vertebra to the affected areas. Acupuncture and moxibustion on related Huatuojiaji points can then be considered as a way to stimulate the nerve pathways, thus potentiating the other points chosen for each treatment.

The girdle vessel can be used to stimulate the flow of qi and blood in the leg channels. For men, the points used are GB 41 (Zulinqi) on the left and SJ 5 (Waiguan) on the right; for women, the sides are reversed. Also, St 36 (Zusanli) and UB 23 (Shenshu) are stimulated to strengthen leg channels.

> If the muscles on the lateral side of the legs are stiff, tonify K 6 (Zhaohai) and reinforce Lu 7 (Lieque), in that order. Reduce UB 62 (Shenmai) and SI 3 (Houxi), in that order.

> If the medial side of the legs is affected, UB 62 (Shenmai) and SI 3 (Houxi) are reinforced; and K 6 (Zhaohai) and Lu 7 (Lieque) are reduced.

Scalp or head acupuncture is increasingly being studied for pain treatments on the extremities, and especially in cases of nerve-related pain. The needle or needles are inserted subcutaneously on a transverse angle of 15° or less to thread the needle to stimulate a large area on either side of the Du/GV channel.

The area of Du/GV 20 (Baihui) is good for neurological degeneration, but it is also helpful for stroke patients with affected limbs. Thread the upper motor area of the scalp for treating the legs and the lower area for the arms.

Bulbar paralysis is related to the Cranial nerves IX-XII (Glossopharyngeal, Vagus, Spinal Accessory and Hypoglossal). Sudhakaran's article goes on to recommend the following points for treating MND with bulbar paralysis presentations:

- For swallowing difficulties, stimulate the needle with an even method on Ren/CV 23 (Lianquan), Ren/CV 24 (Chengjiang), Du/GV 26 (Shuigou), Ren/CV 17 (Danzhong), SI 17 (Tianrong), and LI 18 (Futu); P 6 (Neiguan) and LI 4 (Hegu); and GB 24 (Riyu).

- For excessive salivation, reduce points Ren/CV 23 (Lianquan), Ren/CV 24 (Chengjiang), St 4 (Sanjiao), LI 4 (Hegu), and Sp 9 (Yinlingquan) and St 40 (Fenglong).

- For speech difficulties, even method Ren/CV 23 (Lianquan), Ren/CV 24 (Chengjiang), St 4 (Sanjiao), H 5 (Tongli), and GB 34 (Yanglingquan).

For pattern diagnosis, the following protocols are recommended:

- For St and Sp deficiency, needle St 36 (Zusanli), Sp 3 (Taibai), UB 20 (Pishu), and UB 21 (Weiwhu) and use moxa on Ren/CV 12 (Zhongwan). The herbal formula used is Shenlingbaizhusan (Ginseng, Poria, and Atractylodis Macrocephalae Powder).

- For Liv and K deficiency, reinforce Liv 8 (Ququan), K 3 (Taixi), UB 18 (Ganshu), UB 23 (Shenshu), GB 34 (Yanglingquan), Du/GV 3 (Yaoyangguan), and Ren/CV 4 (Guanyuan). Add formula Huqianwan (Hidden Tiger Pill).

Auricular acupuncture is added to regular acupuncture point treatments and it strengthens the positive outcomes. Sudhakaran suggests testing the following points for tenderness: spinal motor neurons; corresponding body areas; medulla oblongata; brain stem ear shen men point zero; brain; sympathetic autonomic point;

endocrine point; occiput; kidney C; and sanjiao. In her treatment protocol, the ear points that tested positive for pain were stimulated using a Pointer Excel, usually at 10Hz.

As a general note, it is important to state that not all points are used in each session. As always, when you are treating any patient, you must perform a thorough evaluation of their status before, during, and after each session. In any patient that is suffering from debility, chose the least amount of points that foster the greatest amount of benefit.

Acupuncture treatments were given twice per week for eight weeks and then reduced to once monthly for six months. At that point, the pattern was repeated, with twice-weekly treatments for eight weeks, returning to monthly treatments.

MND, and especially MND with bulbar paralysis places patients at a much higher risk of mineral deficiency due to malnutrition. Sublingual treatments are less taxing for these patients than oral medications. For nutritional support, Sudhakaran included mineral salts: 0.5µg (each) of calcium phosphate, potassium phosphate, potassium chloride, magnesium phosphate, and sodium phosphate, given in combination three times per day. She further suggests five drops per day of an alcohol extract of garden daisy (*Bellis perennis*) can be included for its regenerating effects.

The patient was reported to experience considerable symptomatic improvement, to near normalcy; arrest of progression of the disease, evident by the EMG; and slight reduction in the wasting of her muscles. The researcher goes on to state: "Acupuncture cannot have a claim to cure ALS but can be offered with confidence to reduce the symptoms associated with all forms of MND, and improve a patient's quality of life" (Sudhakaran 2017, p.267).

This study is far too limited to make such a claim. Given the early stage of the disease when treated, the duration of treatments, the patient sample size of one, and no long-term follow-up, it does not seem appropriate to generalize the claim to all forms of MND, or all ALS patients. Further studies with larger populations and multiple acupuncturists are needed to validate these findings. However, if you are searching for a place to start a palliative care treatment on a patient with ALS, this material may be helpful.

Can acupuncture help with swallowing difficulties?

As noted previously, a major problem with these conditions is difficulty swallowing, which leads to aspiration, choking, and pneumonia. A study by Vieira *et al.* (2017), while applied to healthy volunteers, may have clinically significant applications for patients who cannot swallow well.

This study measured changes in esophageal motility after acupuncture. The changes of 16 health volunteers (50% females, mean age 26 ± 1.9 years) were measured 20 minutes after acupuncture stimulation of the gastrointestinal point St 36 (Zusanli). Electric stimulation (Accurate Pulse 195 Microprocessor) delivered a dense regular wave with a frequency of 10Hz for 20 minutes. This was adjusted in the first five minutes, with progressive increases in intensity up to the patient's pain threshold, and maintained for 15 minutes more.

The researchers chose St 36 (Zusanli) for its effects in the stomach, to accelerate gastric emptying in patients with gastroparesis, decrease postoperative nausea and vomiting, and stabilize intestinal motility, to treat both diarrhea and constipation.

Lower esophageal sphincter (LES) resting and residual pressure, distal latency (DL), and distal contractility integral (DCI) were recorded. LES resting pressure was significantly reduced after acupuncture. DL was significantly increased after acupuncture as compared to the basal measure. The results showed that acupuncture on the digestive point decreases LES basal pressure and may be an alternative treatment to spastic disorders of the LES.

By treating swallowing and gastrointestinal problems, acupuncture can help patients obtain healthy nutrition and aid in the prevention of cachexia.

Another study (Lee and Kim 2013) focused on the effects of Sa-am acupuncture treatment on the respiratory physiology parameters in ALS patients.

ALS is characterized by progressive neuromuscular atrophy with early involvement of the respiratory system. The latter rapidly leads to pulmonary compromise requiring mechanical ventilation and represents the major cause of mortality. Eighty-four percent of ALS patients die of respiratory complications and respiratory insufficiency in two to three years after diagnosis. However, there is as yet no effective treatment for respiratory dysfunction in ALS patients.

ALS belongs to the category of Wei symptoms in traditional East Asian medicine. The earliest published literature about Wei symptoms is "Plain Question" Treatment in making the digestive system healthy.

In this study, 18 ALS patients received Sa-am acupuncture treatment twice a day for five days. The patients' pulse rate and three measures of respiratory function, end-tidal carbon dioxide ($EtCO_2$), peripheral oxygen saturation (SpO_2), and respiratory rate (RR) were measured for 15 minutes before and during treatment, using capnography and oximetry.

Sa-am acupuncture was conducted at specific acupoints using 0.25 x 40mm, sterile, disposable acupuncture needles made of stainless steel. The depth of insertion for each point was predetermined to be within the normal range of 8–20mm, depending on the location of the point. To tonify lung functions, acupuncture points Sp 3 (Taibai), Lu 9 (Taiyuan), H 8 (Shaofu), and Lu 10 (Yuji) were selected on both sides of the body in accordance with Sa-am Five Element Acupuncture found in the traditional Korean literature. Respiratory muscle weakness and respiratory symptoms such as sputum production and shallow respiration are thought to be related to lung dysfunction.

Sp 3 (Taibai) and Lu 9 (Taiyuan) were employed for tonification of lung qi; H 8 (Shaofu) and Lu 10 (Yuji) were selected to clear lung fire.

The Sp 3 (Taibai) and Lu 9 (Taiyuan) acupoint needles were electrically stimulated at 100Hz with the clinician adjusting intensity so that the patient felt an uncomfortable sensation that was not painful; needles were kept in place for 15 minutes while measuring $EtCO_2$, SpO_2, RR, and pulse rates simultaneously. Each patient received acupuncture treatment twice a day for five days.

The results showed a decrease in $EtCO_2$, RR, and pulse rate and an increase in SpO_2, with significant differences in SpO_2 and pulse rate. Patients in the earlier stages of the disease with high

K-ALSFRS-R scores responded better to acupuncture treatments than the patients with lower K-ALSFRS-R scores. The Amyotrophic Lateral Sclerosis Functional Rating Scale (ALSFRS) is a validated questionnaire-based scale that measures physical functional status in terms of the ability to carry out activities of daily living in patients with ALS.

The study concluded that Sa-am acupuncture treatment on ALS patients seems to be more effective in the early stages of the disease. Treatments appeared to have a greater effect on inspiration rather than on expiration.

Pulmonary disease

Pulmonary disease includes a group of lung diseases that are usually severe and chronic. Chronic obstructive pulmonary disease (COPD), emphysema, bronchitis, cystic fibrosis, tuberculosis, acute respiratory distress syndrome (ARDS), lung cancer, and mesothelioma are the major diseases in this group. More acute and deadly pulmonary diseases include asthma pleural effusion pneumonia, pulmonary embolism (PE), and pneumothorax.

Hospice criteria for pulmonary disease

Patients will be considered to be in the terminal stage of pulmonary disease if they meet the following criteria: 1 and 2 *must* be present; factors 3, 4, and/or 5 provide supporting documentation.

1. Severe chronic lung disease as documented by *both* a and b:

    a. The patient will have disabling dyspnea at rest and poor response or unresponsive to bronchodilators, resulting in decreased functional capacity, e.g. bed to chair existence, fatigue, and cough (documentation of forced expiratory volume in one second (FEV1), after bronchodilator—less than 30% of predicted is objective evidence for severe chronic lung disease, but is not necessary to obtain).

    b. Progression of end-stage pulmonary disease, as evidenced by increasing visits to the emergency department or hospitalizations for pulmonary infections and/or respiratory failure (documentation of serial decreases in FEV1 of greater than 40ml/year is objective evidence for disease progression, but is not necessary to obtain).

2. Hypoxemia, as evidenced by documentation within the last three months of more than one of:

   • Oxygen saturation of 88 percent or less on room air

   • $pO2 \leq 55mmHg$ (these values may be obtained from recent hospital records)

   • Persistent hypercapnia, as evidenced by $pCO2 \geq 50mmHg$ (this value may be obtained from hospital records within the preceding three months).

Documentation of the following factors may provide additional support for end-stage pulmonary disease.

3. Cor pulmonale or right heart failure (RHF) secondary to pulmonary disease (e.g. not secondary to left heart disease or valvulopathy).

4. Unintentional progressive weight loss of greater than 10 percent of body weight over the preceding six months.

5. Resting tachycardia greater than 100 beats per minute.

More information on pulmonary disease

Lung diseases are categorized by the part of the respiratory system that they affect: airways, air sac (alveoli), interstitium, blood vessels, pleura, and chest wall. Smoking, infections, and genetics are the causes of most lung disease. Often, pulmonary disease is tied directly to prolonged exposure to toxic chemicals. The number one cause of preventable pulmonary disease is cigarette smoking. Below is a list of parts of the respiratory system and the diseases that affect them. Notice that some diseases affect more than one level.

   • Airways: asthma, COPD, chronic and acute bronchitis, emphysema, cystic fibrosis

- Alveoli: pneumonia tuberculosis, emphysema, pulmonary edema, lung cancer, acute ARDS, pneumoconiosis (black lung, brown lung, asbestosis)

- Interstitium: interstitial lung diseases, pneumonia, and pulmonary edema

- Blood vessels: pulmonary embolism; pulmonary hypertension

- Pleura: plural effusion, pneumothorax, mesothelioma

- Chest wall: obesity, neuromuscular disorders.

Adapted from Robinson 2019

How can acupuncture help?

As noted in the last study in the neurological disease section of this chapter, tonification of the lung function using Sa-am acupuncture is a valid treatment to help patients with respiration (Lee and Kim 2013). In another randomized, placebo-controlled trial of acupuncture in patients with COPD (Suzuki *et al.* 2012), acupuncture proved to be a promising treatment. The study consisted of 68 patients with dyspnea on exertion (DOE), divided into two groups of 34. One group received real acupuncture, and one group received sham acupuncture (treatment on points unrelated to respiratory functions). Both groups received acupuncture treatments once a week for 12 weeks. After 12 weeks, the Borg scale (a self-reported measure of perceived exertion) score after the six-minute walk test was significantly better in the real acupuncture group compared with the placebo acupuncture group. The study demonstrated that acupuncture is a useful adjunctive therapy in reducing DOE in patients with COPD.

In another study (Cohen, Menter, and Hale 2005), acupuncture has also been shown to reduce breathlessness in cancer patients.

A non-related review of 16 randomized controlled trials, involving 2937 participants, concluded that acupuncture is a safe and potentially effective intervention for patients with asthma and COPD (Jobst 1995). The importance of choosing acupuncture points close to the respiratory accessory muscles was emphasized in the process of determination of the standard treatment. The standardized points used were Lu 1 (Zhongfu), Lu 9 (Taiyuan), LI 18 (Futu), Ren/CV 4 (Guanyuan), Ren/CV 12 (Zhongwan), St 36 (Zusanli), K 3 (Taixi), GB 12 (Wangu), UB 13 (Feishu), UB 20 (Pishu), and UB 23 (Shenshu). The researchers demonstrated clinically relevant improvements in DOE (Borg scale), nutritional status (including BMI), airflow obstruction, exercise capacity, and health-related quality of life after three months of acupuncture treatment (Suzuki *et al.* 2012).

Renal failure

Kidney failure, also called end-stage renal disease (ESRD), is the last stage of chronic kidney disease. The two leading causes of kidney failure are hypertension and diabetes. When the kidneys fail, they are no longer able to filter out waste products from the circulating blood. Water can accumulate in the body if the kidneys cannot function properly to eliminate it. A patient cannot survive without dialysis or a kidney transplant to remove the fluids and toxins that have built up. Over a half million people have kidney disease in the US.

Hospice criteria for renal failure
Patient has 1, 2, and 3:

1. Patient is not seeking dialysis or renal transplant.

2. Creatinine clearance is < 10cc/min (< 15 for diabetics).

3. Serum creatinine is > 8.0mg/dl (> 6.0mg/dl for diabetics).

Supporting documentation for chronic renal failure includes:

- Uremia with obtundation

- Oliguria (urine output < 400cc in 24 hours)

- Intractable hyperkalemia (> 7.0)

- Uremic pericarditis
- Hepatorenal syndrome
- Intractable fluid overload.

Supporting documentation for acute renal failure includes:

- Mechanical ventilation
- Malignancy (another organ system)
- Chronic lung disease
- Advanced cardiac disease.

Supporting documentation of comorbidities:

- History of mechanical ventilation
- Malignancy (another organ system)
- Chronic lung disease
- Advanced cardiac disease
- Advanced liver disease
- Sepsis
- Immunosuppression/AIDS
- Albumin cachexia
- Platelet count < 25,000
- Disseminated intravascular coagulation
- Gastrointestinal bleeding.

Diabetes is the most common cause of ESRD. High blood pressure is the second most common cause of ESRD. Other problems that can cause kidney failure include:

- Autoimmune diseases, such as lupus and IgA nephropathy
- Genetic diseases (diseases you are born with), such as polycystic kidney disease

- Nephrotic syndrome

- Urinary tract problems.

Sometimes the kidneys can stop working very suddenly (within two days). This type of kidney failure is called acute kidney injury or acute renal failure. Common causes of acute renal failure include:

- Heart attack

- Illegal drug use and drug abuse

- Not enough blood flowing to the kidneys

- Urinary tract problems.

This type of kidney failure is not always permanent. Your kidneys may go back to normal or almost normal with treatment and if you do not have other serious health problems.

Having one of the health problems that can lead to kidney failure does not mean that you will definitely have kidney failure. It is essential for the patient to live a healthy lifestyle.

Chronic kidney disease (CKD) usually gets worse slowly, and symptoms may not appear until your kidneys are badly damaged. In the late stages of CKD, nearing kidney failure (ESRD), the patient may experience the following symptoms as metabolic waste and extra fluid accumulate in the body:

- Itching

- Muscle cramps

- Nausea and vomiting

- Not feeling hungry

- Swelling in feet and ankles

- Too much urine (pee) or not enough urine

- Trouble catching their breath

- Trouble sleeping.

If the kidneys stop working suddenly (acute kidney failure), they may notice one or more of the following symptoms:

- Abdominal (belly) pain

- Back pain

- Diarrhea

- Fever

- Nosebleeds

- Rash

- Vomiting.

One or more of any of these symptoms may be a sign of kidney failure. The patient should contact a physician or go to the emergency department immediately.

Patient profile

Chronic kidney disease can affect any population, but there are risk factors that make some people more susceptible to development of the disease. Some of these factors are preventable, such as diabetes (Type 2), hypertension, cardiovascular disease, smoking, and obesity. Other factors that add to the risk of kidney disease are genetic; for instance, African-American, Native American, and Asian-American populations tend to have higher numbers of people affected. Also, a family history of kidney disease, or abnormal kidney structure or polycystic kidney disease, puts an individual at higher risk. As kidney qi declines, older-aged people are more inclined to have kidney disease.

There are cultural and nutritional factors that can add to the risk. In countries where schools and jobs have become more sedentary and more stress inducing, hypertension has increased in the general populations. Add in the fact that fast foods and junk foods with high fructose corn syrup, high sodium, and high saturated fats have become readily available not only in every corner market, or drive-thru restaurant, but just down the hall in the break area (even in hospitals), and obesity has become endemic. The patient with chronic hypertension will be prescribed medicine that is known to damage the kidneys, often diabetes follows, and with it, chronic kidney disease.

Acupuncture in renal failure

Once again, the diseases that can lead to end-stage renal disease, namely diabetes and hypertension, respond well to acupuncture, therapeutic diet, and herbal medicine. During a typical treatment, 6 to 12 points are needled for 20–30 minutes. Commonly used points are: St 36 (Zusanli), Sp 6 (Sanyinjiao), UB 23 (Shenshu), Ren/CV 6 (Qihai), and UB 20 (Pishu). During the treatment, other points can be added according to symptoms and signs. A recent study (Cui *et al.* 2013) on essential hypertension recommended one point as the most effective: K 3 (Taixi).

Uremic pruritus (a severe and persistent itching skin that can lead to sleeplessness and mood disorder) is a common problem in end-stage renal failure patients. In one study (Che-yi *et al.* 2005), acupuncture was tested for hemodialysis patients at the LI 11 (Quchi) acupoint for refractory uremic pruritus. There were 40 patients who were randomly divided into two groups of 20. Acupuncture was applied unilaterally at LI 11 (Quchi) for the first group. The second (control) group received acupuncture on a non-point, 2cm from LI 11 (Quchi). Each patient received three treatments per week for one month, for a total of 12 treatments.

The patients completed a questionnaire before the treatments started, at the end of the month of treatments, and again at a three-month follow-up session. Participants gave scores for itching, distribution of locations, and sleep disturbance. Pruritus scores were graded and compared. Both groups started at a score of 38.3 + 4.3, but the control group scores only dropped by about 1 point, whereas the acupuncture group dropped to 17.3 + 5.5 at the end of the first month, and 16.5 + 4.9 at the three-month follow-up session. These findings are statistically significant. The good news for your patients is that acupuncture at LI 11 (Quchi) is an easy, safe, and effective means of relieving uremic pruritus. Imagine how many lives you could change if this technique was included in a community-style acupuncture model in a dialysis clinic.

Acupuncture for renal function

In another study, on the effects of acupuncture on renal function in patients with chronic kidney disease (Yu *et al.* 2017), 59 subjects were divided into two groups. The first group of 30 participants received regular acupuncture; the control group of 29 received sham acupuncture.

Acupuncture was applied bilaterally to LI 4 (Hegu), St 36 (Zusanli), and K 3 (Taixi) to obtain qi, and electroacupuncture (2Hz) was applied to both the right and left pairs of St 36 (Zusanli) and K 3 (Taixi), once per week, for 12 weeks for the first group. The control group received acupuncture, but subcutaneously on the same three point groups, and no electrostimulation.

Patients' serum creatinine levels and eGFRs (estimated glomerular filtration rates) were measured at the start of the study, after the 12 weeks of treatment, and at a three-month follow-up. Of the 53 patients who completed the treatments, there were changes in the average scores of both groups, but much more pronounced change in the first group. Acupuncture at bilateral LI 4 (Hegu), St 36 (Zusanli), and K 3 (Taixi) for 12 weeks reduced creatinine levels and increased eGFR levels. The conclusion was that this is a feasible model for the treatment of patients with chronic kidney disease.

Stroke or coma

A stroke occurs when the blood supply to part of the brain is interrupted or reduced, depriving brain tissue of oxygen and nutrients. The most common cause of strokes is a clot in the blood vessels leading to or around the brain. It is the fifth highest cause of death and a leading cause of disability in the US. A stroke can lead to a coma. A coma is a deep state of prolonged unconsciousness in which a person cannot be awakened, fails to respond normally to painful stimuli, light, or sound, lacks a normal wake-sleep cycle, and cannot initiate voluntary actions.

Hospice criteria for stroke or coma

Patients will be considered to be in the terminal stage of stroke or coma if they meet the following criteria. For stroke, criteria 1 and 2 are important indicators of functional and nutritional status and will support a terminal prognosis for patients with a diagnosis of stroke; 3 will lend support.

1. Poor functional status with a Palliative Performance Scale (PPS) of 40 or less. All criteria here should be met:

   - Mainly bedbound

   - Unable to work

   - Requires maximal assistance to perform self-care

   - Food/fluid intake are normal/reduced

   - Either fully conscious or drowsy/confused

   AND

2. Inability to maintain hydration and caloric intake with *one* of the following:

   - Weight loss > 10 percent during previous six months

   - Weight loss > 7.5 percent in previous three months

   - Serum albumin

   - Current history of pulmonary aspiration without an effective response to speech language pathology interventions to improve dysphagia and decrease aspiration events

   - Calorie counts documenting inadequate caloric/fluid intake

   - Dysphagia severe enough to prevent the patient from receiving food/fluid that is necessary to sustain life in a patient who does not receive artificial nutrition/hydration.

3. Documentation of medical complications within the previous 12 months, in the context of progressive clinical decline, will help support eligibility for hospice care.

- Recurrent or intractable infections such as pneumonia or other respiratory tract infection

- Urinary tract infection

- Sepsis

- Refractory stage 3–4 decubitus ulcers

- Fever recurrent after antibiotics.

The medical criteria listed below would support a terminal prognosis for individuals with a diagnosis of coma (any etiology). Comatose patients with any three of the following on day three of their coma are considered terminal:

- Abnormal brain stem response

- Absent verbal response

- Absent withdrawal response to pain

- Serum creatinine > 1.5mg/dl.

More information on stroke and coma

There are five types of stroke:

- Ischemic: from clots blocking the flow of blood to the brain; these account for 87 percent of all strokes.

- Hemorrhagic: caused by bleeding from the rupture of a weakened blood vessel.

- Trans ischemic attacks (TIAs): often called mini-strokes, and derive from a temporary blockage of blood flow to the brain. These strokes are considered to be a warning sign that a major stroke is possible.

- Cryptogenic: the origin of the stroke cannot be found.

- Brain stem: happen in the brain stem, as opposed to the brain. These strokes are very serious and leave the patient unable to speak, or move below the neck.

In the emergency department when they talk about a stroke they say, "Time equals brain," meaning the less time between the on-set of symptoms and initial treatment, the better the outcome. Signs and symptoms of a stroke should be timed from when the first indication begins. The length of time also changes treatment options. A person having a stroke can experience:

- trouble with speaking and understanding. Confusion, slurring words, or difficulty understanding speech can happen

- paralysis or numbness of the face, arm, or leg. This often happens on one side of the body. To assess, have the person raise both arms straight out and try to maintain that hold while they close their eyes. If one or both arms drift or drop, that is a sign. If the mouth droops when they try to smile, or if one cheek and the skin around an eye appear lower than the other side, seek immediate help

- trouble with seeing in one or both eyes. The person may suddenly experience blurred vision or black spots in their vision, or they may see double

- headache. A sudden, severe headache, which may be accompanied by vomiting, dizziness, or altered consciousness, may indicate a stroke. Patients often describe this as the worse headache of their life

- trouble with walking. If the person stumbles, lists to one side, or experiences sudden dizziness, loss of balance, or loss of coordination, seek immediate help.

Patients who suffer a stroke or a coma are first at risk for losing their lives, or at least the function of part or parts of their brain and/or bodies. Second, stroke and coma conditions simply leave patients vulnerable to dying from some sort of infection, malnutrition, dehydration, or pneumonia. Once a person is physically disabled and movement is severely restricted, then circulation and respiration suffer. Every beginning student of Asian Medicine knows that if you want to move qi, move blood, and yet in order to move blood most efficiently, the body itself must move.

Muscles that cannot contract make swallowing much more difficult. This alone can cause a person to lose weight. When attempting to eat a normal meal becomes a struggle, or when every liquid requires a thickening agent to keep the person from gagging, it can lead to anorexia.

If the epiglottis does not close automatically, food or saliva can enter the trachea and cause choking or lead to particles of food entering the lungs and possibly causing aspiration pneumonia. Furthermore, if that person has a limited gag or cough response, they may not be able to rid their body of the resulting phlegm, and therefore choke to death.

There may be bladder problems as well. The bladder may not signal it is full, or the ability to urinate to drain the bladder completely may be missing. Waste materials then build up, leading to bladder infection, or, in worse-case scenarios, the ureters and then the kidneys can become infected, and if the kidney function is decreased, then blood does not get filtered, leading to possible sepsis, or chronic or acute kidney failure.

Of course, there are antibiotics to help fight infections, but frequent use of antibiotics can lead to decreased intestinal bacteria, and that can further affect digestion. The other side effect of frequent antibiotics is that they become less effective, as bacteria can mutate and form super strands that are resistant to antibiotic treatment. There are times in the hospice treatment where doctors will simply stop prescribing antibiotics.

Decubitus ulcers, also commonly called bedsores, are a problem seen in bedbound, chair-bound, or minimally active patients. Thin patients are often at a higher risk, as the fat pad between bone and skin is minimal, or missing. Preventative care requires the patient to turn, or be repositioned, every two hours as prolonged pressure causes the circulation to decrease in the affected area, and that leads to tissue death or damage.

What causes a coma?

A coma is a prolonged state of unconsciousness. During a coma, a person is unresponsive to their environment. The person is alive and looks as if they are sleeping. However, unlike in a deep sleep, the person cannot be woken by any stimulation, including pain.

Comas are caused by an injury to the brain. Brain injury can be due to increased pressure, bleeding, loss of oxygen, or build-up of toxins. The injury can be temporary and reversible. It also can be permanent. More than 50 percent of comas are related to head trauma or disturbances in the brain's circulatory system. The following are problems that can lead to coma:

- *Trauma*: Head injuries can cause the brain to swell and/or bleed. When the brain swells as a result of trauma, the fluid pushes up against the skull. The swelling may eventually cause the brain to push down on the brain stem, which can damage the reticular activating system (RAS)—a part of the brain that is responsible for arousal and awareness.

- *Swelling*: Swelling of brain tissue can occur even without distress. Sometimes a lack of oxygen, electrolyte imbalance, or hormones can cause swelling.

- *Bleeding*: Bleeding in the layers of the brain may cause coma due to swelling and compression on the injured side of the brain. This compression causes the brain to shift, causing damage to the brain stem and the RAS. High blood pressure, cerebral aneurysms, and tumors are non-traumatic causes of bleeding in the brain.

- *Stroke*: When there is no blood flow to a major part of the brain stem or loss of blood accompanied with swelling, coma can occur.

- *Blood sugar*: In people with diabetes, coma can occur when blood sugar levels stay very high. That's a condition known as hyperglycemia. Hypoglycemia, or blood sugar that is too low, can also lead to a coma. This type of coma is usually reversible once the blood sugar is corrected.

- *Oxygen deprivation*: Oxygen is essential for brain function. Cardiac arrest causes a sudden cut-off of blood flow and oxygen to the brain, called hypoxia or anoxia. After cardio-pulmonary resuscitation (CPR), survivors of cardiac arrest are often in comas. Oxygen deprivation can also occur with drowning or choking.

- *Infection*: Infections of the central nervous system, such as meningitis or encephalitis, can bring on a coma.

- *Toxins*: Substances that are normally found in the body can accumulate to toxic levels if the body fails to dispose of them correctly. For example, ammonia due to liver disease, carbon dioxide from a severe asthma attack, or urea from kidney failure are all toxic to the body in higher levels. Drugs and alcohol in large quantities can also be toxic to the liver or kidneys, and disrupt neuron functioning in the brain.

- *Seizures*: A single seizure rarely produces coma. Continuous seizures called status epilepticus have been known to bring on a coma. Repeated seizures can prevent the brain from having recovery time between seizures, leading to prolonged unconsciousness and coma.

Acupuncture for strokes and coma

There is some discussion about when treatment for a stroke should begin. Some practitioners are in favor of waiting a couple of weeks in the case of ischemic strokes. There are many studies in Japan, China, and Korea that show acupuncture is beneficial as an adjunct to Western medical treatments for stroke.

If you could only pick one point to needle on a patient after a stroke, consider GB 34 (Yanglingquan). This point is used to help recover motor function in stroke patients and is accompanied by increased neural activities in motor-related brain regions (according to neuroimaging studies). GB 34 (Yanglingquan) may increase motor cognition connectivity, including visual memory, motor task learning, and motor intention. These functions help patients recover from hemiplegia and spasm (Association of Traditional Chinese Medicine & Acupuncture 2015).

According to a discussion narrated by Dr. Yu-ning Lin (2008), of Tzu Chi General Hospital:

> Strokes, cerebral embolisms, cerebral hemorrhages, and brain injuries…can be treated with acupuncture. In China, a combination with modern imaging techniques of the cerebral cortex, and treatments that combined scalp and body pressure points, are employed to treat coma patients. As with all coma and stroke-related treatments, the earlier an appropriate procedure begins, the better the results and the lower the rates of disability in the patients. (Lin 2008)

Dr. Yu-ning Lin goes on to explain that benign stimuli (scalp points) can bring about an "awakening" of the brain. Body acupuncture then plays two roles: through the spinal cord, it excites the cells of the paralyzed muscle to prevent atrophy; and repeated stimulus near the peripheral receptors can stimulate nerve cells in unaffected areas, incessantly sending the stimulus brought forth by the needle point, where this signal is transmitted to the central nervous system to excite the brain, and, in turn, signal it to repair the neurons.

He does not mention specific points; the practitioner would have to know the areas affected to choose the correct protocol. He does conclude that the function of acupuncture is mainly to increase muscle strength, ease tension and stiffness, and reduce abnormal reflexes. Given the description of the bio-physiology of the c-fibrin discussed earlier in the book in the section on how acupuncture works, the practitioner should be advised to select points that stimulate the largest possible sections of the affected areas.

Other acupuncture subjects that are relative to the care of stroke and coma patients are included in the neurological disease section regarding aspiration precautions, and the terminal illness section on the care of bedbound patients.

Terminal illness: general (non-specific)

General terminal illness (non-specific) is most commonly seen in the frail elderly who may not have one of the specific hospice diagnoses discussed above, but may have one or more chronic illnesses. In the absence of a known terminal illness, these patients often have poor appetite, loss of weight, increased fatigue, and a progressive functional decline. Such frail elders may be eligible for the services provided by the Medicare Hospice Benefit.

Hospice criteria for terminal illness

Patients with this diagnosis have a terminal condition not attributed to a single illness, *and* rapid decline over the past three to six months, as evidenced by:

- decline in PPS to < 50 percent

- involuntary weight > 10 percent and/or albumin < 2.5 (helpful)

- progression of disease evidenced by signs, symptoms, and test results.

The medical criteria below support the terminal prognosis for patients with adult failure to thrive syndrome. Criteria 1 and 2 *must* be met; factor 3 will lend support to terminal status. The patient would meet criteria if *all* of the following are met.

1. Irreversible nutritional impairment, as evidenced by both of the following:

   - Body Mass Index (BMI) will be less than $22kg/m^\wedge$ (BMI $(kg/m^\wedge 2) = 703x$ (weight in pounds) / (height in inches) $^\wedge 2$)

   - Declines enteral/parenteral nutritional support, OR has not responded to such support, despite an adequate caloric intake

   AND

2. Significant disability as evidenced by the Palliative Performance Scale (PPS) **equal to or less than 40 percent.**

3. Other variables lending support to terminal diagnosis include the following:

- Recurrent or intractable infections, such as pneumonia or other upper respiratory infection (URI), sepsis, or UTI

- Decreasing serum albumin or cholesterol

- Dysphagia leading to recurrent aspiration and inadequate oral intake documented by the decreasing food portion consumption

- Nausea/vomiting, poorly responsive to treatment

- Diarrhea, intractable

- Generalized pain

- Decline in systolic blood pressure to below 90 or progressive postural hypotension

- Edema

- Change in level of consciousness

- Abnormal electrolyte levels

- Progressive 3–4 stage pressure ulcers.

More information on terminal illness

This diagnosis was previously labeled "adult failure to thrive" (AFTT), or "debility, not otherwise specified." Now, physicians are directed to "Identify the condition that is the main contributor to the person's terminal prognosis." Non-specific diagnoses such as AFTT may no longer be listed as a principal terminal diagnosis. Debility and AFTT can and should be listed as secondary (related) conditions to support prognosis if indicated. These changes in clinical variables apply to patients whose decline is not considered to be reversible. They are examples of findings that generally connote a poor prognosis.

The hospice physician is responsible for determining the diagnosis or diagnoses that are the most likely cause of the patient's terminal prognosis. In some cases, a single diagnosis, such as pancreatic cancer, accurately describes the basis for that prognosis. In others, there may be related diagnoses, for example Alzheimer's dementia and aspiration pneumonia. Finally, there are some cases in which multiple prognosis-determining diagnoses combine to give the patient a prognosis of less than six months, for example ischemic cardiomyopathy and chronic obstructive pulmonary disease. There are numerous methods used to determine the prognosis; one not previously discussed is the Karnofsky Performance Status (KPS) (Péus, Newcomb, and Hofer 2013; see Table 9.2). Much like the PPS, it measures the patient's overall ability to maintain a normal activity level.

Initially, study of the KPS showed that performance status is an important predictor of survival. Further work has attempted to refine the ability to predict length of survival. Pre-existing disease, prior treatment, psychological status, and social support may affect the length of survival in a terminal illness.

Table 9.2: Karnofsky Performance Scale percentage criteria

100	Normal; no complaints; no evidence of disease
90	Able to carry out normal activity; minor signs or symptoms of disease
80	Normal activity with effort; some signs of symptoms of disease
70	Cares for self; unable to carry on normal activity or do active work
60	Requires occasional assistance, but is able to care for most of his/her needs
50	Requires considerable assistance and frequent medical care
40	Disabled; requires special care and assistance
30	Severely disabled; hospitalization is indicated, although death not imminent
20	Very sick; hospitalization necessary, active supportive treatment necessary
10	Moribund; fatal processes progressing rapidly
0	Dead

The PPS is a modification of the KPS, designed specifically for measurement of the physical status of the patient, with additional descriptions regarding eating and specifics around sleep. Using the PPS, only about 10 percent of patients with a score of 50 percent or less would be expected to survive more than six months. Other studies have used clinical symptoms along with performance scales.

The Palliative Prognostic Index (PPI) is an example of such a tool, using the PPS along with oral intake, edema, dyspnea at rest, and delirium. Unlike other predictors, the lower the number, the better the prognosis. The patient scores zero if everything is normal; with 15 being the worst score. If the patient's PPI is greater than 6, survival is less than three weeks; greater than 4 it is six weeks; and less than 4, the patient has longer than six weeks to live.

One prognostic score, the PaP (Palliative Prognostic Score), includes use of anorexia, dyspnea, total white blood count, and lymphocyte percentage along with the KPS and expert clinical prediction of survival. Based on the results of these variables, patients are considered to belong to one of three prognostic groups, reflecting 30-day survival probability of > 70 percent, 30–70 percent, or < 30 percent.

Patient profile

Failure to thrive speaks for itself; this is not the normal aging process, but rather a combination of age with other disease influences. The patients often present with multiple symptoms, including, but not limited to, weight loss (usually with signs of reversible nutrition deficiency, even after attempts at supplement nutrition), anorexia, dehydration, depression, and impaired immune function. Poor nutrition and inadequate hydration mean the body has no reserves to sustain life. Many times, these patients often have bladder and bowel problems that result in diarrhea or constipation (often complicated with impactions). Patients may be mentally and physically disabled.

In common language, these patients are often "nothing but skin and bones." The body has a natural wisdom that communicates to the mind it is simply worn out, and the organs are no longer able to function at a level that maintains life. There is no official terminal illness; they may be dying from a cascade effect, leading to multiple organ or system failure. In Asian Medicine terms, it is the depletion of yin and yang. Often the stomach qi becomes so diminished that food is no longer appealing or capable of being processed. Once the stomach stops acquiring nutrients, the rest of the organ functions are so far out of balance they override one another.

Patients who have limited mobility, or who are chair- or bedbound for any amount of time (especially those with no fat pad), are at special risk for skin tears and decubitus ulcers (commonly called bedsores). Prevention of these problems requires special handling of the frail patient, which includes turning the patient slowly and carefully every two hours to prevent prolonged pressure to one area of the body. Patients who are incontinent must be checked, cleaned, and changed to prevent bacteria that can lead to infection or further skin breakdown. A combination of pillows, pads, egg-crate mattresses, and air-circulating mattresses may also be employed in the effort to prevent or lessen the damage to a patient's skin.

Acupuncture for terminal illness

Bedsores are rated by their severity, with stage I being an area of redness, and stage IV being so deep it may affect ligaments or muscles. In stage II sores, skin is broken, leaves an open wound, or looks like a pus-filled blister. The area is swollen, warm, and/or red, and it is difficult to determine the exact depth and border. The sore may ooze clear fluid or pus, and it's painful.

In stage III, the sores have gone through the second layer of skin into the fat tissue. The sore has a crater-like appearance and often has a bad odor. It may show signs of infection: red edges, pus, odor, heat, and/or drainage. There may be black, necrotic (dead) tissue in or around the sore.

In one acupuncture study (Yang *et al.* 2017), bedsores were treated with the turtle technique. There were 34 patients who all had stage II and III sores. Seventeen patients were in each group. Prior to treatment, the wound area in both groups was cleaned with 3 percent hydrogen peroxide solution and 0.9 percent sodium chloride solution. Next, in a sterile environment, blisters were pierced to drain inflammatory secretions and to debride the wound.

One treatment group received acupuncture plus standard wound care. The other group received only standard wound care. Fire acupuncture was used at the wound site. Needles were heated to a red-hot state, inserted, and withdrawn at the fastest speed possible, to a depth of 5–10mm.

Next, a surround acupuncture procedure was applied. A total of four 0.03mm x 40mm disposable needles were obliquely inserted surrounding each ulcerative lesion. Each needle was distal to the lesion by 1cm. After that, an electroacupuncture device was connected to the acupoints. A disperse-dense wave (750μA, 0.5Hz) was applied with an intensity level set to patient tolerance levels or until muscle contractions were observable. Needles were retained for 15 minutes once the electroacupuncture stimulation was initiated.

Finally, a TDP (Teding Diancibo Pu) heat lamp was applied for 10 minutes at a 25–30cm distance from the ulcerative lesions. The lamp was set to patient tolerance levels.

These treatments were given once per day, five days per week, for a total of three weeks, and 15 treatments.

The results were based on the wound measurements at the end of the three weeks. Patients receiving acupuncture plus standard wound care had an 88.2 percent effective rate. The control group who did not receive acupuncture, only standard wound care, had a 70.6 percent total effective rate. It must be noted that these patients may not have been terminal, so they may have an added bonus of still being able to ingest healing nutrients. Furthermore, a Kennedy terminal ulcer is not in this category—it generally appears 48 hours before death, and cannot be cured.

Chinese herbs for infection and sepsis

Sepsis is one of the top ten causes of disease-related deaths. Bodies with weak or compromised immune systems can overreact to an infection, or simply not be able to fight off bacteria. Septicemia is a bacterial infection in the blood, which leads to sepsis. Poisons are released by the bacteria into the bloodstream. Once the blood is poisoned, the circulating toxins can infect other tissues and organ systems, leading to multi-organ failure and, inevitably, death.

Recently, researchers at the Feinstein Institute for Medical Research in the US have discovered that the humble and simple mung bean used in Traditional Chinese Medicine can help with infection and sepsis. In technical terms, it reduces the release of HMGB1 (a nucleosomal protein that has recently been established as a late mediator of lethal systemic inflammation), which in theory can increase survival rates by slowing the reproduction of bacteria (Lade 2013). The beans can be sprouted or used in a soup and processed in a blender for people who are experiencing problems with solid foods.

The last treatment

Finally, the Hospice Acupuncture Protocol described in Chapter 7 of this book can be used to help ease the physical, spiritual, and emotional pain of the dying patient. It is important to remember that, on particularly frail patients, needling can lead to fainting, so please exercise your best clinical judgment and utilize acupressure or non-contact energetic stimulation when treating fragile patients. Always treat your patients with care and respect. Remember to speak to them with kindness, as if your words may be the last words they ever hear…you never know.

Conclusion

First, let me address the obvious. Scientific research and new medications are an ongoing part of the overall picture of healthcare. There are new strides being made every day in the understanding, treating, curing, and eradicating of diseases. Where Asian Medicine has focused on the treatment of the individual and bringing the patient back to balance, Western medicine is now leaning to more personalized/individualized treatments based on DNA, and making remarkable strides in turning a person's immune system back on to essentially cure from within. This may be the beginning of the tipping point for the human race. Indeed, in the not so distant future, the leading causes of death could be from the effects of war, environmental changes, and overpopulation, rather than disease processes.

We must focus on the present, but be mindful of our effects for the future. For acupuncturists, that means we must continue to practice, to teach our patients about nutrition, exercise, and self-care. We must employ Asian Medicine to bring them back into balance so that they have the best chance of living lives free of symptoms of disharmony and debilitating disease. We must continue to push for insurance coverage, so that we might serve a larger segment of the population. We must educate our patients, the general population, and the current medical system in all the ways that we know to help and heal, with all the modalities that are available in our scope of practice.

So how do we get hospice acupuncture covered by insurance? We must be approved by Medicare. In essence, we have to provide skilled care for a problem, and, generally, that skill has to be backed up with hard scientific research and studies. As a profession, we have to come together to pool our collected efforts and to highlight our true worth. Although it is wonderful that we know, for instance, that acupuncture helps people with nausea and vomiting from the effects of chemotherapy, we must gather larger pools of indisputable data to showcase our other treatment outcomes. So how do we do that?

One possible gateway for consolidating studies is the World Health Organization (WHO). Many practitioners use the WHO's list to find out and advertise what acupuncture has been approved for, but how many practitioners are either participating in a WHO research project, or turning over the results of their studies with others? There is a richness of wisdom and opportunities available on the WHO website under the complementary and integrative medicine headings.

It is an indisputable fact that, sooner or later, everyone on the face of this earth dies. It has been happening for millions of years, and, unless we make this planet too toxic or environmentally hostile to live on, it will continue to happen.

In hospice circles, there is often a joke that goes "Life is a terminal condition." Death is an age-old, natural process. And yet, when a person is stricken with an illness that is known to be "terminal," we often hear language from medical professionals, family members, friends, and/or the patient about fighting this illness together.

Somewhere along the way, when we took death away from the family home, we stopped having essential conversations about it.

There is a common belief, despite millions of years of evidence to the contrary, that it is somehow more noble to "go down fighting." This appears to be a bizarre double-standard around death. Perhaps this comes from our war-torn past where young men were encouraged to heal by not giving up. To die peacefully without a fight sometimes leads to hushed, shamed whispers (i.e. "She didn't even try to take dialysis, or chemotherapy"). As if subjecting yourself to a known toxic process which leaves you vomiting with no energy is somehow valued and expected.

Hospice and palliative care strive to support the person in their vision of death, not ours. If a patient wants to fight a disease using every experimental drug available so they might gain an extra month of life, that is their choice; they may have to be discharged from the hospice, but they can be reinstated when heroic methods no longer work. If a person decides they have seen the end, and they want to opt out of weeks of not being able to walk to the bathroom, or being in unrelenting pain, or losing the ability to swallow their favorite treat, then that choice is theirs as well.

We are there to help the patient in their desire. We are also there to support and educate the family or circle of care. Family members may try to prolong a person's life by force-feeding them. The body has an innate wisdom, and if a person wants to stop eating, they should not be forced to eat. This can end up in vomiting or aspiration pneumonia. First do no harm should apply to all caregivers, be they professionals or laypeople.

There are ethical dilemmas that we must solve personally and as a society. Much like a baby under "normal circumstance" can be born and expect to survive, a person with a terminal illness under normal circumstances is expected to die. And as a mother may be induced into labor, making the birth predictable, the dying patient in some places may be allowed to have a physician-assisted "suicide," thus giving the patient control of their dying circumstances. Perhaps the suicide name (and thus, the stigma) should be removed all together. The disease is what kills the patient, the physician or medication is just a means of moving the process of death to its natural end.

When a person cannot walk, talk, eat, drink, or otherwise function, one must ask, just because we have the technology to keep them alive, should we use it? Conversely, just because we have the means to terminate the patient's life, should we use it? That's why those medical directives are so very important.

Chapter 10

Final Thoughts

As a member of a hospice interdisciplinary team you have a multifaceted role. You must study and learn about hospice and palliative care so you can present yourself as a competent practitioner. You are telling the public that there is a special skill set that should be expected and asked for when patients are being treated at the end of life. Using your knowledge and experiences, you must educate hospice team members about the potential use of Asian Medicine in hospice care, and support them by sharing information about the patients you are caring for.

Remember that your role is to move qi and help the dying patient release physical, emotional, and spiritual blocks to ease the dying process. Treat your patients and their loved ones with dignity and respect. Never lose sight of these people as whole beings—they are much more than their behaviors, situations, or ailments. Be open to broadening your own vision by listening to others who have shared their life stories. If you embrace this rewarding work, you will be touched in ways you cannot yet imagine. Some people call hospice workers "midwives for death." Death, like birth, is a profoundly sacred act and you may be the privileged witness to the end of a life cycle.

Dame Cicely Saunders put it so well: "You matter because of who you are. You matter to the last moment of your life, and we will do all we can, not only to help you die peacefully, but also to live until you die" (2011).

NAHPCA Treatment Protocol

Patient Name: _____ Date: __/ __/__

Location: _____ Time: _____AM PM

Tongue: _____Tongue coating: _____

Pulse Rate: before TX ____ after TX ____

Heart Rate: before TX____ after TX____

Respiration rate: before TX____ after TX____

Pain level:

before TX 0 1 2 3 4 5 6 7 8 9 10

after TX   0 1 2 3 4 5 6 7 8 9 10

Notes: _____

_____

_____

_____

_____

_____

_____

Patient is currently expressing:

Denial Anger Bargaining   Depression   Acceptance

Have patient rate emotional state on a scale of 0–5, where 0 is none, 3 is problematic, and 5 is unbearable.

Wood: Anger, injustice about dying

0 1 2 3 4 5

Fire: Despair, loneliness, isolation, contracted spirit, feeling unlovable

0 1 2 3 4 5

Earth: Obsession, self-absorption, worry, anxiety, victimized

0 1 2 3 4 5

Metal: Denial, not accepting, refusal to let go of life

0 1 2 3 4 5

Water: Fear, survival issues

0 1 2 3 4 5

Other issues/emotions or voiced concerns:

_____

_____

_____

_____

_____

_____

NAHPCA Points	Right	Left	Bilateral	Electrostimulation	Moxa
WOOD					
☐ Liv 3	☐	☐	☐	☐	☐
☐ Liv 13	☐	☐	☐	☐	☐
☐ Liv 14	☐	☐	☐	☐	☐
☐ GB 40	☐	☐	☐	☐	☐
FIRE					
☐ H 1	☐	☐	☐	☐	☐
☐ H 7	☐	☐	☐	☐	☐
☐ SI 11	☐	☐	☐	☐	☐
☐ P 3	☐	☐	☐	☐	☐
☐ P 4	☐	☐	☐	☐	☐
☐ P 6	☐	☐	☐	☐	☐
☐ P 7	☐	☐	☐	☐	☐
☐ SJ 4	☐	☐	☐	☐	☐
☐ SJ 7	☐	☐	☐	☐	☐
☐ SJ 10	☐	☐	☐	☐	☐
EARTH					
☐ Sp 3	☐	☐	☐	☐	☐
☐ Sp 6	☐	☐	☐	☐	☐
☐ Sp 21	☐	☐	☐	☐	☐
☐ St 36	☐	☐	☐	☐	☐
☐ St 40	☐	☐	☐	☐	☐
☐ St 42	☐	☐	☐	☐	☐
METAL					
☐ Lu 1	☐	☐	☐	☐	☐
☐ Lu 3	☐	☐	☐	☐	☐
☐ Lu 7	☐	☐	☐	☐	☐
☐ Lu 9	☐	☐	☐	☐	☐
☐ LI 4	☐	☐	☐	☐	☐
☐ LI 11	☐	☐	☐	☐	☐
☐ LI 17	☐	☐	☐	☐	☐
☐ LI 18	☐	☐	☐	☐	☐

cont.

NAHPCA Points	Right	Left	Bilateral	Electrostimulation	Moxa
WATER					
☐ K3	☐	☐	☐	☐	☐
☐ K 20	☐	☐	☐	☐	☐
☐ K 21	☐	☐	☐	☐	☐
☐ K 23	☐	☐	☐	☐	☐
☐ K 24	☐	☐	☐	☐	☐
☐ K 25	☐	☐	☐	☐	☐
☐ UB 44 (39)	☐	☐	☐	☐	☐
☐ UB 47 (42)	☐	☐	☐	☐	☐
☐ UB 52 (47)	☐	☐	☐	☐	☐
☐ UB 57	☐	☐	☐	☐	☐
☐ UB 61	☐	☐	☐	☐	☐
☐ UB 64	☐	☐	☐	☐	☐
Special/Other					
☐ Ren/CV 14					
☐ Du/GV20					
☐ Sishencong					
☐_____					
☐_____					
☐_____					
Total Needle Count:					

Practitioner's Signature_____

Glossary for Point Nomenclature

Please note that this list only includes the points from Chapter 8. This glossary is only meant to be a handy referral guide, and is not meant to replace proper education or clinical training. The use of point selection is the sole responsibility of the licensed practitioner. The following terms are an attempt to be inclusive of the diversity of terminology in acupuncture texts and teachings. In most incidences, the Chinese name will be listed first.

Ancestor points (unofficial term) help to get the patient in touch with ancient archetypes and those who have gone before. SI 11 (Tianzong), SJ 7 (Sanjiao), Du 20 (Baihui).

Crossing/Coalescent/Points of Intersection are located where two or more of the 12 regular and eight extra channels or meridians intersect. They may be used to treat disorders that appear simultaneously on their intersecting channels. Liv 13 (Zhangmen)—Gallbladder; Liv 14 (Qimen)—Spleen and Yin Linking Channel; Sp 6 (Sanyinjiao)—Three Leg Yin/Kidney and Liver; Lu 1 (Zhongfu)—Spleen; K 20 (Tonggu)—Chong; K 21 (Youmen)—Chong; UB 61 (Pucan)—Yangwei and Yangqiao; Du 20 (Baihui)—Urinary Bladder (but also known as Crossing Point of All Yang Channels).

Eight Xi/Confluent/Opening/Meeting Points of the Eight Extraordinary/Miscellaneous Channels link the 12 regular channels and the eight extraordinary channels. They are mainly Yuan and Luo points—found on the upper or lower limbs. These points treat symptoms related to their respective regular channel.

P 6 (Neiguan)—Yin Wei/Linking Channel; Lu 7 (Lieque)—Ren/ Conception (Sea of Yin) Channel.

Entry points are where energy enters the channel or meridian. H 1 (Jiquan), Lu 1 (Zhongfu), LI 4 (Hegu).

Exit points are where energy leaves the channel or meridian. Liv 14 (Qimen), St 42 (Chongyang), Lu 7 (Lieque).

General Connecting point: While Sp 21 (Dabao) is the regular connecting point on the Spleen Channel; its original luo connectiong point is Sp 4 (Gongsun). Although Sp 4 (Gongsun) is noteworthy, it is not part of the hospice protocol. All four extremities acquire vital energy indirectly from the stomach with the help of the spleen.

The stomach sends fluids to the five zang organs and the four limbs through the spleen's major collateral.

Hui/Gathering/Meeting/Eight Influential points regulate the zang-fu organs and are where the qi of their respective body tissues (blood, tendons, vessels, bones and marrow) are infused into the body surface. Liv 13 (Zhangmen)—zang/yin organs; Lu 9 (Taiyuan)—vessels.

Lower He/Sea points are where the qi of yang channels travels downward and accumulates. They enhance communication between all yang channels. St 36 (Zusanli)—Sea of Food/Grains (Stomach).

Luo/Connecting points can be used alone to treat full or empty symptoms of each connecting channel. A connecting point can also be used in conjunction with the source point of its interior-exterior related channel to treat disorders of its organ. It reinforces the action of the source point, which works as the main point for treating the primarily affected channel. P 6 (Neiguan), Sp 21 (Dabao), St 40 (Fenglong), Lu 7 (Lieque).

Mother/Reinforcing/Tonification points are stimulated to increase the flow of qi within the channel/meridian and its related organ system. Lu 9 (Taiyuan), LI 11 (Quchi).

Mu/Front/Alarm/Collecting points are located on the chest and abdomen (hence the name Front-Mu points) in close proximity to their respective zang-fu organs. Mu points are where the qi of the relevant organs is infused and collects or gathers. They become sensitive or tender—either with pressure from touch, or spontaneously when their respective organ is diseased—hence the "Alarm" title. Liv 13 (Zhangmen)—Spleen; Liv 14 (Qimen)—Liver; Lu 1 (Zhongfu)—Lungs; Ren 14 (Juque)—Heart.

Sea of Marrow point increases mental functioning and energy levels. When the sea is deficient, a person may experience fatigue, tinnitus, weakness in the lower limbs, and so on. Du 20 (Baihui).

Sedation/Reducing/Son points are used to reduce excess syndromes. These are part of the mother and son combinations. H 7 (Shenmen), P 7 (Daling), SJ 10 (Tianjing).

Shu/Transporting/Command/Element points are found between fingers and elbows, and toes and knees. These points represent the growth of qi in the channels as it ascends up the limbs. They include the following:

- **Shu/Stream/Transporting points** are where qi pours through and the channels and defensive qi gathers. These points are used for sensations like heaviness, dampness, and joint pain. Liv 3 (Taichong), H 7 (Shenmen), P 7 (Daling), Sp 3 (Taibai), Lu 9 (Taiyuan), K 3 (Taixi).

- **He/Sea/Uniting points** are where the course of the superficial distal channels moves inward and centripetal to their deep proximal courses, where qi is vast and slow. These points are used for rebellious qi and diarrhea. P 3 (Quze), SJ 10 (Tianjing), St 36 (Zusanli), LI 11 (Quchi).

Spirit points (unofficial term) have a spirit name that is heavily relied on to decide which point is appropriate for the patient. Usually, these points are chosen from the patient's causative factor channel/meridian. Tonify a point holding the Spirit of the Point in mind and summoning that energy from the point. Your intention when needling should match the intention of the point.

K 20 (Futonggu), K 21 (Youmen), K 23 (Shenfeng), K 24 (Lingxu), K 25 (Shencang), UB 44 (39) (Shengteng), UB 47 (42) (Hunmen), UB 52 (47) (Zhishi).

Window to the Sky points improve the flow of qi between the body and the head by "opening the window." Lu 3 (Tianfu), LI 18 (Futu).

Wu Xing/Five Phases/Movements/Element points

- **Tu/Earth points** treat dampness and phlegm. Liv 3 (Taichong), H 7 (Shenmen), P 7 (Daling), SJ 10 (Tianjing), Sp 3 (Taibai), St 36 (Zusanli), Lu 9 (Taiyuan), LI 11 (Quchi), K 3 (Taixi)

- **Shui/Water points** treat cold. On yin channels, it is the He/Sea point; on yang channels, it is the Ying/Spring point. P 3 (Quze).

Xi/Cleft/Accumulation points are where the qi of the channel gathers. These points move stagnant qi and are mostly used in acute patterns and to dispel pain. P 4 (Ximen), SJ 7 (Huizong).

Yuan/Primary/Source point energy stems from deep levels of original qi and is related to the yin organs, especially the kidneys. Source points are used to tonify yin organs on the yin channels. The yang organ source points are mostly used in excess patterns to expel pathogenic factors. Liv 3 (Taichong), GB 40 (Qiuxu), H 7 (Shenmen), P 7 (Daling), SJ 4 (Yangchi), Sp 3 (Taibai), St 42 (Chongyang), Lu 9 (Taiyuan), LI 4 (Hegu), K 3 (Taixi), UB 64 (Jinggu).

References

Albright, M.A. (2006) "How China gives hospice care: Local nurse learns how similar we are." *Corvallis Gazette Times*, December 6. Accessed on 06/12/06 at www.gazettetimes.com/articles/2006/11/09/news/community/4aa04_hospice.txt.

American Cancer Society (2009) *What is hospice care?* Accessed on 19/11/09 at www.cancer.org/docroot/ETO/content/Eto_2_5x_What_Is_Hospice_Care.asp.

Anderson, F., Downing, G.M., Hill, J., Casorso, L., and Lerch, N. (1996) "Palliative Performance Scale (PPS): A New Tool." *Journal of Palliative Care*, 12(1), 5–11.

Anastasi, J., Chang, M., Capili, B., and Dawes, N. (2011) "Traditional Chinese Medicine and human immunodeficiency virus-associated neuropathy." *Journal of Chinese Medicine*, 95(2), 16–20.

Association of Traditional Chinese Medicine & Acupuncture (2015) *Acupuncture Treatment for Stroke*. London: Association of Traditional Chinese Medicine & Acupuncture. Accessed on 05/05/19 at www.atcm.co.uk/acupuncture-treatment-for-stroke

Brassington, D. (1998) *Spirit of the Points (Excluding the Bladder Meridian) Version 2*. Baltimore, MD: TAI Sophia.

British Acupuncture Council (2012) *Acupuncture and HIV Infection*. London: British Acupuncture Council. Accessed on 15/05/18 at https://static1.squarespace.com/static/547db623e4b036ff1df2a3b6/t/548f11fde4b03d9f5cd9d5e7/1418662397798/HIV_november_2012.pdf.

British Acupuncture Council (2014) *Neuropathic Pain*. London: British Acupuncture Council. Accessed on 08/09/18 at www.acupuncture.org.uk/a-to-z-of-conditions/a-to-z-of-conditions/neuropathic-pain.html.

Centers for Disease Control and Prevention (2016) "*QuickStats*: Percentage Distribution of Deaths, by Place of Death—United States, 2000–2014." *Morbidity and Mortality Weekly Report (MMWR)* 65, 357. DOI: http://dx.doi.org/10.15585/mmwr.6513a6.

Centers for Disease Control and Prevention (2017) "Deaths and Mortality." *National Center for Health Statistics.* Accessed on 09/19/19 at https://www. cdc.gov/nchs/fastats/deaths.htm.

Chan, C.L.W. and Chow, A.Y.M. (eds) (2006) *Death, Dying and Bereavement: A Hong Kong Chinese Experience.* Hong Kong: Hong Kong University Press.

Chang, B., Boehmer, U., Zhao, Y., and Sommers, E. (2007) "The combined effect of relaxation response and acupuncture on quality of life in patients with HIV: A pilot study." *Journal of Alternative and Complementary Medicine,* 13(8), 807–815.

Chang, B. and Kemp, C. (2003) *Refugee health ~ Immigrant health: Chinese.* Accessed on 20/11/09 at https://web.archive.org/web/20140720092817/ https://bearspace.baylor.edu/Charles_Kemp/www/chinese.htm.

Chang, B. and Sommers, E. (2011) "Acupuncture and the relaxation response for treating gastrointestinal symptoms in HIV patients on highly active antiretroviral therapy." *Acupuncture Medicine,* 29(3), 180–187.

Che-yi, C., Cheng, Y., Kao, M., and Huang, C. (2005) "Acupuncture in haemodialysis patients at the Quchi (LI11) acupoint for refractory uraemic pruritus." *Nephrology Dialysis Transplantation,* 20(9), 1912–1915. DOI: 10.1093/ndt/gfh955.

China Daily (2006) "Chinese still reluctant to place loved ones in hospice." *China Daily,* April 6. Accessed on 15/12/09 at http://en.people. cn/200604/06/eng20060406_256395.html.

Cohen, A.J., Menter, A., and Hale, L. (2005) "Acupuncture: Role in comprehensive cancer care—a primer for the oncologist and review of the literature." *Integr Cancer Ther,* 4(2), 131–143.

Connor, S. and Bermedo, M. (eds) (2014) *Global Atlas of Palliative Care at the End of Life.* Geneva: World Health Organization; Worldwide Palliative Care Alliance, pp.35–41. Accessed on 05/04/19 at www.who.int/nmh/ Global_Atlas_of_Palliative_Care.pdf.

Council of Colleges of Acupuncture and Oriental Medicine (2009) *Know your acupuncturist.* Accessed on 05/12/09 at www.ccaom.org/downloads/ KnowYourAcupuncturist.pdf.

Cui, S., Xu, M., Wang, S., Tang, C., Lai, X., and Fan, Z. (2013) "Antihypertensive effect of acupuncturing at KI3 in spontaneously hypertensive rats." *2013 IEEE International Conference on Bioinformatics and Biomedicine,* Shanghai, 19–25. DOI: 10.1109/BIBM.2013.6732747.

Deng, G., Vickers, A., D'Andrea, G., Xiao, H., *et al.* (2007) "Randomized, controlled trial of acupuncture for the treatment of hot flashes in breast cancer patients." *Journal of Clinical Oncology,* 12(35), 5584–5590.

Denver Hospice (2009) *Complementary therapies.* Accessed on 13/12/09 at https://thedenverhospice.org/our-services/integrative-therapies.

Department of Health and Human Services (2018) *Centers for Medicare and Medicaid Services: Hospice Medicare Benefits.* Washington, DC: Department of Health and Human Services. Accessed on 04/06/19 at www.medicare.gov/pubs/pdf/02154-medicare-hospice-benefits.pdf.

DerSarkissian, C. (reviewer) (2019) *The Stages of Cancer According to the TNM System*. New York: WebMD Medical References. Accessed on 05/05/19 at www.webmd.com/cancer/cancer-stages?print=true.

Dharmananda, S. (1999) *The treatment of ALS with Chinese Medicine*. Accessed on 21/05/09 at www.itmonline.org/arts/als.htm.

Dogin, M. (ed) and New York Heart Association, Criteria Committee (1994) *Nomenclature and Criteria for Diagnosis of Diseases of the Heart and Great Vessels*, 9th ed. Boston, MA: Little, Brown and Company.

Felman, A. (2018) "Explaining HIV and AIDS." *Medical News Today*. Accessed on 10/08/18 at www.medicalnewstoday.com/articles/17131.php.

Filshie, J. and Rubens, C. (2011) "Acupuncture in palliative care." *Acupuncture in Medicine*, 29(3), 166–167.

Flaws, B. (1995) *The Secret of Chinese Pulse Diagnosis* (pp.132–133). Boulder, CO: Blue Poppy Press.

Fox, L. (2010) *Palliative Performance Scale*. Kingston: Queens University Faculty of Health Sciences. Accessed on 09/18/19 at www.collaborative curriculum.ca/en/modules/PPS/PPS-thepalliativeperformancescale-01.jsp.

Garcia, M., McQuade, J., Haddad, R., Patel, S., *et al.* (2013) "Systematic review of acupuncture in cancer care: A synthesis of evidence." *Journal of Clinical Oncology*, 31(7), 952–960.

Harrison, I. (2008) *Hospice care*. Cancer Supportive Care Programs National and International. Accessed on 13/12/09 at www.cancersupportivecare.com/hospice.html#Philosophy.

Health CMi (2015) *Acupuncture Benefits Alzheimer Disease Patients*. Capitola: Healthcare Medical Institute. Accessed on 06/05/18 at www.healthcmi.com/Acupuncture-Continuing-Education-News/1491-Acupuncture-Continuing-Education-News/1491-acupuncture-benefits-alzheimer-disease-patients.

Health CMi (2016a) *Acupuncture plus herbs alleviate cirrhosis and ascites*. Accessed on 05/05/18 at www.healthcmi.com/Acupuncture-Continuing-Education-News/1627-acupuncture-plus-herbs-alleviate-cirrhosis-and-ascites.

Health CMi (2016b) *Acupuncture Alleviates Angina, Beats Drugs on EKG*. Capitola: Healthcare Medical Institute. Accessed on 08/09/18 at www.healthcmi.com/Acupuncture-Continuing-Education-News/1675-acupuncture-beats-drugs-for-ekg.

Hopkins Technology (1995) *Fever due to impairment of internal organs*. Acupuncture.com. Accessed on 06/08/18 at www.acupuncture.com/Conditions/feverzf.htm.

Hospice and Palliative Care of Virginia (2009) *History of Hospice*. Informational Paper. Norton: Hospice and Palliative Care of Virginia.

Hospice Association of America (2009) *Hospice: An HAA/NAHC Historical Perspective*. Handout. Washington, DC: Hospice Association of America Facts and Statistics, Hospice Forum, Caring Magazine.

Hospice by the Bay (2018) *Determining a patient's prognosis of six months or less for hospice.* Accessed on 08/05/18 at http://hospicebythebay.org/resources/lcd-and-physician-letter-3-15-16.pdf.

Hospice Minnesota for Care of the Dying (2009) *People to people: A life changing experience.* Accessed on 05/12/09 at https://www.hospicevolunteer association.org/HVANewsletter/0160_Vol3No2_2007Apr06_PTPinChina Tibet-LifeChangingExperience.pdf.

Hospice of Michigan (2009) *Brief history of the hospice movement.* Accessed on 15/12/09 at https://web.archive.org/web/20070702151025/http://www.hom.org/movement.asp

Jobst, K.A. (1995) "A critical analysis of acupuncture in pulmonary disease: Efficacy and safety of the acupuncture needle." *J Altern Complement Med,* 1(1), 57–85.

Kanakura, Y., Niwa, K., Kometani, K., and Nakazawa, Y. (2002) "Effectiveness of acupuncture and moxibustion treatment for lymphedema following intrapelvic lymph node dissection: A preliminary report." *The American Journal of Chinese Medicine,* 30(1), 37–43.

Kasymjanova, G., Grossman, M., Tran, T., Jagoe, R., *et al.* (2013) "The potential role for acupuncture in treating symptoms in patients with lung cancer: An observational longitudinal study." *Current Oncology,* 20(3), 152–157.

Kaufman, K. and Salkeld, E.J. (2008) "Home hospice acupuncture: A preliminary report of treatment delivery and outcomes." *The Permanente Journal,* 12(1), 23–26.

Kübler-Ross, E. (1969) *On Death and Dying.* New York: Scribner.

Lade, H. (2013) *Chinese herbs and infection for sepsis.* The Acupuncture Clinic. Accessed on 08/06/18 at www.theacupunctureclinic.co.nz/chinese-herbs-for-infection-and-sepsis.

Lafferty, W.E., Tyree, P.T., Devlin, S.M., Anderson, R., and Diehr, P.K. (2008) "Complementary and alternative medicine provider use and expenditures by cancer treatment phase." *The American Journal of Managed Care,* 14(5), 326–334.

Laino, C. (2005) *Acupuncture eases side effects of AIDS drugs: People report less bloating, cramping.* WebMD Archives.

Lee, M. (1992) *Insights of a Senior Acupuncturist.* Boulder, CO: Blue Poppy Press.

Lee, S. and Kim, S. (2013) "The effects of Sa-Am acupuncture treatment on respiratory physiology parameters in amyotrophic lateral sclerosis patients: A pilot study." *Evidence-Based Complementary and Alternative Medicine.* Accessed on 05/05/19 at www.hindawi.com/journals/ecam/2013/506317.

Leng, G. (2013) "Use of acupuncture in hospices and palliative care services in the UK." *Acupuncture in Medicine,* 31(1), 16–22.

Li, J., Li, J., Chen, Z., Liang, F., Wu, S., and Wang, H. (2012) "The influence of PC6 on cardiovascular disorders: A review of central neural mechanisms." *Acupuncture in Medicine,* 30(1), 47–50.

Liangyue, D., Yijun, G., Shuhui, H., Xiaoping, J., *et al.* (1987) *Chinese Acupuncture and Moxibustion.* Beijing: Foreign Language Press.

Lin, Y. (narr.) (2008) "From coma to consciousness: Not a miracle." *Medicine with Humanity*, 9(5), 50–51.

Lynch, T., Connor, S., and Clark, D. (2013) "Mapping levels of palliative care development: A global update." *Journal of Pain and Symptom Management*, 45(6), 1094–1106.

Maciocia, G. (1989) *The Foundations of Chinese Medicine: A Comprehensive Text for Acupuncturists and Herbalists.* Philadelphia, PA: Elsevier.

Master Travel Limited (part of The Mark Allen Group) (2005) *Reflections on a study tour to China.* Accessed on 20/11/09 at https://web.archive.org/web/20090305153310/www.mastertravel.co.uk/articles.php?article=10.

McPhail, P., Sandhu, H., Dale, J., and Stewart-Brown, S. (2018) *Acupuncture in hospice settings: A qualitative exploration of patients' experiences.* Accessed on 11/03/18 at https://onlinelibrary.wiley.com/doi/abs/10.1111/ecc.12802.

Melbourne Zen Hospice (2009) *Introducing acupuncture.* Accessed on 11/12/09 at https://web.archive.org/web/20090510063458/http://www.zen.org.au/acupuncture.html.

Mitchell, T. (2017) *The Leading Causes of Death in the World – Can They Be Cured?* London: ProClinical. Accessed on 08/08/18 at www.proclinical.com/blogs/2017-5/the-leading-causes-of-death-in-the-world-can-they-be-cured.

National Hospice and Palliative Care Organization (2009a) *Hospice FAQs.* Accessed on 13/12/09 at www.nhpco.org/hospice-care-overview/hospice-faqs.

National Hospice and Palliative Care Organization (2009b) *Keys to quality care.* Accessed on 13/12/09 at https://web.archive.org/web/20131221171156/http:/www.nhpco.org/about-hospice-and-palliative-care/keys-quality-care.

National Hospice and Palliative Care Organization (2017) *Facts and Figures: Hospice Care in America.* Alexandria: National Hospice and Palliative Care Organization. Accessed on 12/03/19 at https://www.nhpco.org/wp-content/uploads/2019/07/2018_NHPCO_Facts_Figures.pdf.

National Hospice and Palliative Care Organization (2019) *History of hospice care.* Accessed on 05/05/19 at https://www.nhpco.org/hospice-care-overview/history-of-hospice.

National Institute of Health (2016) *World's Population Grows Dramatically: NIH-funded Census Bureau report offers details of global aging phenomenon.* Bethesda: NIH…Turning Discovery Into Health. Accessed on 12/09/19 at www.nih.gov/news-events/news-releases/worlds-older-population-grows-dramatically.

Nieminen, T. (2001) *Acupuncture and Chinese Medicine: Roleplaying in Asian settings 4*, December 19. Accessed on 20/11/09 at https://web.archive.org/web/20090503161225/www.qugs.org.au/queensland-wargamer.

Pajka, S. (2017) *Doctors, Death, and Denial: The Origins of Hospice Care in 20th Century America.* New Haven: Yale University EliScholar – A Digital Platform for Scholarly Publishing at Yale. Accessed on 09/18/19 at https://pdfs. semanticscholar.org/5795/477dc77931132e8f913bfb7a096bb091245b.pdf.

Péus, D., Newcomb, N., and Hofer, S. (2013) "Appraisal of the Karnofsky Performance Status and proposal of a simple algorithmic system for its evaluation." *BMC Medical Informatics and Decision Making 13*(72). Accessed on 05/05/19 at https://bmcmedinformdecismak.biomedcentral. com/articles/10.1186/1472-6947-13-72#Sec12.

Price, C. (2011) *Enhancing xenobiotic detox.* Naturopathic Doctor News and Review, December 2011. Accessed on 24/05/19 at https://ndnr.com/pain-medicine/liver-acupuncture.

Puhky, R. (2001) "Five Element acupuncture for terminal patients: A powerful intervention for dying well." *Medical Acupuncture: A Journal for Physicians by Physicians,* 12(1), 32–37.

Reisberg, B. (1988) "Functional Assessment Staging (FAST)." *Psychopharmacology Bulletin,* 24, 653–659.

Ritchie, H. and Roger, M. (2019) "Causes of death." *Our World in Data.* Accessed on 07/06/19 at https://ourworldindata.org/causes-of-death.

Robinson, J. (reviewer) (2019) "Lung diseases overview." *WebMD Medical Reference.* Accessed on 05/05/19 at https://www.webmd.com/lung/lung-diseases-overview#1.

Romeo, M.J., Parton, B., Russo, R.A., Hays, L.S., and Conboy, L. (2015) "Acupuncture to treat the symptoms of patients in a palliative care setting." *Explore,* 11(5), 357–362. Accessed on 03/04/18 at www.explorejournal. com/article/S1550-8307(15)00108-1/fulltext.

Saunders, C. (2011) *The Problem of Euthanasia (Care of the Dying-1).* Oxford: Oxford University Press. Accessed on 09/18/19 at https://www. oxfordscholarship.com/view/10.1093/acprof:oso/9780198570530.001.0001/ acprof-9780198570530.

Schwartz, M. (2009) Staff training registration form (unpublished training materials). Denver, CO: The Denver Hospice.

Seladi-Schulman, J. (2019) "What Are the Stages of Liver Failure?" *Healthline Media.* Accessed on 05/05/19 at https://www.healthline.com/health/liver-failure-stages.

Shanghai College of Traditional Medicine. (1981) *Acupuncture: A Comprehensive Text.* Trans. J. O'Connor and D. Bensky. Seattle, WA: Eastland Press.

Shiflett, S. and Schwartz, G. (2011) "Effects of acupuncture in reducing attrition and mortality in HIV-infected men with peripheral neuropathy." *Explore,* 7(3), 148–154.

Soh, K. (2004) "Bonghan duct and acupuncture meridian as optical channel of biophoton." *Journal of the Korean Physical Society,* 45(5), 1196–1198.

St. John, T. (2002) "Chronic Hepatitis B and C in China." *Hepatitis Magazine* (2002, Spring). Accessed on 20/11/09 at https://web.archive.org/web/20100927094559/http://hepcchallenge.org/pdf/chronic%20hepatitis%20in%20china_article_reformat1006.pdf.

Standish, L.J., Kozak, L., and Cogdon, S. (2008) "Acupuncture is underutilized in hospice and palliative care." *American Journal of Hospice and Palliative Care Medicine*, 25(4), 298–308.

Stanrock, J. (2007) *A Topical Approach to Life-Span Development*. New York: McGraw-Hill.

Strong, K., Mathers, C., Leeder, S., and Beaglehole, R. (2005) "Preventing chronic diseases: How many lives can we save?" *The Lancet*, 366 (9496), 1578–1582.

Sudhakaran, P. (2017) "Amyotrophic lateral sclerosis: An acupuncture approach." *Medical Acupuncture*, 29(5), 260–268.

Suzuki, M., Muro, S., Ando, Y., *et al.* (2012) "A randomized, placebo-controlled trial of acupuncture in patients with chronic obstructive pulmonary disease (COPD): The COPD Acupuncture Trial (CAT)." *Archives of Internal Medicine*, 172(11), 878–886.

Therrien, A. (2018) *Alternative cancer therapies linked to reduced survival*. London: BBC News. Accessed on 04/03/19 at www.bbc.co.uk/news/health-44884601.

UNAIDS (2018) *2030: Ending the AIDS Epidemic*. Fact sheet. Accessed on 24/05/19 at www.unaids.org/sites/default/files/media_asset/UNAIDS_FactSheet_en.pdf.

United States Census Bureau (2009) *Facts for features & special editions: Oldest baby boomers turn 60!* Accessed on 23/11/09 at www.census.gov/Press-Release/www/releases/archives/facts_for_ features_special_feditions/006105.html.

United States Census Bureau (2019) *U.S. and World Population Clock*. Accessed on 09/19/19 at https://www.census.gov/popclock.

Unschuld, P. (1998) *Forgotten Traditions of Ancient Chinese Medicine: A Chinese View from the Eighteenth Century. The i-hsueh yuan liu lun of 1757 by Hsu Ta-ch'un*. Taos, NM: Paradigm Publications.

Vieira, F.M., Herbella, F.A.M., Habib, D.H., and Patti, M. (2017) "Changes in esophageal motility after acupuncture." *Journal of Gastrointestinal Surgery*, 21(8), 1206–1211.

Vlasto, T. (2018) *New Scientific Breakthrough Proves Why Acupuncture Works*. San Francisco, CA: American College of Traditional Chinese Medicine at California Institute of Integral Studies. Accessed on 05/05/19 at www.actcm.edu/blog/acupuncture/new-scientific-breakthrough-proves-why-acupuncture-works.

Wang, J. and Zou, W. (2010) "Recent advances of HIV/AIDS treatment with traditional Chinese medicine in China." *Journal of Traditional Chinese Medicine*, 30(4), 305–308.

Wong, M. (2007) *How traditional Chinese health beliefs and Chinese culture influence health and illness?* Ezine, December 13. Accessed on 13/12/09 at http://ezinearticles.com/?id=903741.

World Health Organization (2003) *Acupuncture: Review and analysis reports on controlled clinical trials.* Geneva: World Health Organization. Accessed on 08/05/19 at http://digicollection.org/hss/en/d/Js4926e/7.html.

World Health Organization (2018a) *Palliative Care.* Geneva: World Health Organization. Accessed on 21/10/18 at www.who.int/news-room/fact-sheets/detail/palliative-care.

World Health Organization (2018b) *Cancer.* Geneva: World Health Organization. Accessed on 21/01/18 at www.who.int/news-room/fact-sheets/detail/cancer.

Xie, H. (2011) *How to use acupuncture for the treatment of heart failure.* World Small Animal Veterinary Association World Congress Proceedings Paper. Gainesville: College of Veterinary Medicine, University of Florida.

Xu, L., Xu, H., Gao, W., Wang, W., Zhang, H., and Lu, D. (2013) "Treating angina pectoris by acupuncture therapy." *Acupuncture Electrotherapy Research*, 38(1–2), 17–35.

Yang, J., Wei, Q., Xu, Z., Li, J., *et al.* (2017) "Observations of the efficiency of acupuncture plus TDP in treating stage II–III pressure sores." *Shanghai Journal of Acupuncture and Moxibustion*, 36(5), 568–572.

Yao, C., Tang, N., Xie, G., Zheng, X., *et al.* (2012) "Management of hepatic encephalopathy by Traditional Chinese Medicine." Hindawi Publishing Corporation. *Evidence Based Complementary and Alternative Medicine.* Accessed on 08/08/18 at http://dx.doi.org/10.1155/2012/835686.

Yu, J., Ho, C., Wang, H., Chen, Y., and Hseih, C. (2017) "Acupuncture on renal function in patients with chronic kidney disease: A single-blinded, randomized, preliminary controlled study." *Journal of Alternative and Complementary Medicine*, 23(8), 624–631. DOI: 10.1089/acm.2016.0119.

Zhang, C., Bian, J., Meng, Z., Meng, L., *et al.* (2016) "Tongguan Liqiao acupuncture therapy improves dysphagia after brainstem stroke." *Neural Regeneration Research*, 11(2), 285–291.

Index

abdomen, diagnostic
changes 72, 75
abdominal cramps 67, 95,
101, 143, 145, 149, 154,
178
acceptance of dying 64
accreditation of hospices
19–20
"active dying" 56
acupressure, with children
74
acupuncture
aims of 33
diagnostic investigations
65–79
explanation for how it
works 51–3
fees and insurance cover
54–5, 195
measurement of effects
51–2
neuroscience of 51–3
number of treatments
needed 54
research and effectiveness
studies 35, 55, 58–61
training and education 32
treatable conditions 58–60
use of needles 53–4
uses in palliative and
hospice care 57–61
in Western cultures 32–4,
34–5
see also acupuncture use
with the dying
acupuncture meridians see
acupuncture points and
meridians (overview)

acupuncture needles see
needles
acupuncture points and
meridians (overview)
diagnostic changes 75
and the Five Elements 91
functions and indications
(overview) 51
Hospice Acupuncture
Protocol points 10, 61,
86–91, 201–4
neuroscience of 51–3
treatment points
nomenclature 205–8
treatment techniques and
protocols 86–91, 201–4
acupuncture use with the
dying 57–61
benefits of use 85
frequency of use 85
hospice protocols for use
10, 61, 86–91, 201–4
needle insertions 86
for resolving emotional
conflicts 82–91
treatment techniques 86
Alarm points 207
Albright, M.A. 29
alcohol abuse 110
Alzheimer's disease 131
studies on acupuncture use
133–4
American Cancer Society
14, 37
amyotrophic lateral sclerosis
(ALS) 163
patient profiles 164–5
use of acupuncture 166–9
and Wei symptoms 171–2

Anastasi, J. 148
ancestor points 87–8,
99–100, 205
for anger feelings 90
for negative feelings and
fears 89
Anderson, F. 38
anger feelings 64
and the Wood Element 83,
88, 93–4
angina pectoris, studies on
acupuncture use 137–8
animal therapies 45–6
anorexia 122, 184, 191–2
antibiotic use 184
anxieties 95–7
and the Earth Element
83–4
appetite 72–3
aromatherapy 46
art therapy 46
Asian Medicine
cultural factors 25–7
effectiveness of 31–2, 34–5
hospice and palliative care
10–11, 28–30
key approaches 33
obstacles to inclusion
10–11
scope of 31–2, 33
studies 122–7, 148–50,
154–61
and Western Medicine
31–2
see also TCM (Traditional
Chinese Medicine)
Association of Traditional
Chinese Medicine &
Acupuncture 186–7

asthenia syndromes 126
auricular acupuncture
    160–1, 168–9

baby boomers 9–10
    demographic data 9–10
    need for hospice care
        9–10, 40
Baihui (Du / GV 20) 112–13,
    205, 207
bargaining behaviors 64
bedsores 69, 184, 192–3
bereavement services 39
Bermedo, M. 18
bipolar presentations 97
bladder problems 184
Blood Connecting Channels,
    diagnostic changes 69–70
blurred vision 72
the body, diagnostic changes
    66
body smells 71
Bonghan channels 52–3
bowel movements 73
Brassington, D. 93
breath, changes to 71
breathing
    changes in 70
    and spiritual connections
        83
    terminal stages of dying
        70, 83
    treatments 109
    see also pulmonary disease
British Acupuncture Council
    148–9, 165–6
Buddhism, burial practices
    28
bulbar paralysis 168–9
burials, cultural practices
    27–8

calmness and relaxation
    95–7
cancer
    clinical findings 116–17
    common forms of 118
    common symptoms of
        122–3
    comorbidities 117
    hospice criteria 116–17
    morbidity data 118
    refusal of conventional
        treatments 126–7

stages of 120
studies on use of
    acupuncture 121–7
candidiasis 143
cardiovascular disease see
    heart disease
causes of death (US) 40–1
CD4 cells 141
Centers for Disease Control
    and Prevention 39
Centers for Medicare and
    Medicaid Services (CMS)
    21–2
    on "terminal illness"
        criteria 57
C fibers 51–2
Chan, C.L.W. 28
Chang, B. 26–9, 148–9
Channels (overview) 205–6
    diagnostic changes 69–70,
        73
    therapeutic use of 93–112
    see also acupuncture
        points and meridians
        (overview)
chaplains 43–4
chemotherapy, acupuncture
    in treatment of nausea/
    vomiting 121
Chengshan (UB 57) 111
Che-yi, C. 179
Cheyne-Stokes breathing 70
children
    concepts of death 74
    use of alternative
        treatments 74
chills and fevers 72, 94,
    125–6
China
    funding for care 29
    healthcare system 31–2
    hospice and palliative care
        28–30
    life expectancy 29
    population data 29
    population health and
        disease profiles 29–30
    post-death beliefs and
        rituals 27–8
    role of the family 26–8
    search for longevity 25–6
    see also Asian Medicine
China Daily 25, 28–9
choking 184

Chongyang (St 42) 102–3,
    206
Chow, A.Y.M. 28
chronic non-infectious
    diseases, China 29–30
chronic obstructive
    pulmonary disease
    (COPD)
    use of acupuncture studies
        174–5
    see also pulmonary disease
Clark, D. 9
Cleft / Accumulation points
    208
climate qi, and the Five
    Elements 91
Coalescent points 205
Cogdon, S. 60
Cohen, A.J. 174
Collecting / Mu points 207
colors, and the Five
    Elements 91
coma
    causes of 185–6
    hospice criteria 181–2
    use of acupuncture studies
        186–7
comorbidities 78
complementary therapies,
    and survival rates 126–7
Conception: Ren points 113
Connecting / Luo points 206
Connor, S. 9, 18
cor pulmonale 173
costs of hospice care 19
coughing 70–1
Council of Colleges of
    Acupuncture and
    Oriental Medicine 42
creative or expressive arts 46
Crossing points 205
cryptosporidosis 143
Cui, S. 179
cyanosis 67, 69

Dabao (Sp 21) 101, 206
Daling (P 7) 98–9, 138,
    207–8
dampness and phlegm 91,
    100, 102, 106, 158, 207,
    208
deafness 73
death
    causes of (US) 40–1
    time of 83

death and dying
   bodily changes 66–70,
      70–1, 71–4, 74–5, 75–9
   cultural practices and
      beliefs 9, 29, 30, 67–8,
      195–6
   see also dying process
"death rattle" 70
dehydration 191–2
demeanor, diagnostic
   changes 66
dementia 128–34
   forms of 131
   hospice criteria for 128–30
   patient profiles 131–3
   research on acupuncture
      use 133–4
Deng, G. 124
denial feelings 64–5
   and the Metal Element 83
Denver Hospice 45–7
Department of Health and
   Human Services 57
depression 64, 98
"de qi" 54
despair, and the Fire Element
   84
Dharmananda, S. 163, 165
diabetes
   and liver disease 153
   non-insulin dependent
      137, 176, 178–9
   and renal failure 176,
      178–9
diagnosis giving 190
   and adult failure to thrive
      (AFTT) 189–90
diagnostic investigations
   65–78
   feeling and touch 74–5
   hearing and smelling 70–1
   listening to the patient's
      experiences 71–4
   observations 65–70
   pulse diagnosis 75–9
diarrhea 73, 112–13, 122,
   142–3, 145, 148–50, 170,
   191, 207
disclosure of prognosis, in
   Chinese cultures 27
dizziness 66, 72, 97, 98, 102,
   106, 112–13
dry mouth, treatment studies
   123–4

dying process
   Five Element treatments
      81–91
   the last treatment 194
   talking about 27, 195–7
   see also terminal illness
dyspnea (shortness of
   breath) 33, 59–60, 72,
   172

ear acupuncture 160–1,
   168–9
ears, diagnostic changes 68
Earth Element (obsessions
   and anxieties) 83–4
   channel points 100–3, 203
education and training
   for acupuncture
      practitioners 32, 42
   for patients and family 39
ehospice 22
Eight Influential points 206
Eight Xi Channels 205–6
ejection fraction (EF)
   measures 136–7
electroacupuncture 160
"Elixir of Life" 25–6
emotional issues
   surrounding dying
   Five Element resolution of
      conflicts 82–4, 91
   stages of grief and loss
      63–5
emotional repression 104–5
emotional scales (NAHPCA
   protocol) 202
end-stage renal disease
   (ESRD) see renal failure
energy levels 95, 206–8
   treating deficiencies 99,
      101–2, 103, 112–13,
      133, 207
energy medicine 46
entry points 206
essential hypertension 179
exit points 206
eyes, diagnostic changes 67

facial changes see head and
   face
facial flushes, treatment
   studies 124
family-based care
   in China 26–8

support for caregivers 38–9
   in the US 39–40
fear about dying
   acupuncture points 88,
      89–90
   and the Water Element
      82–3
fees and care charges 21
Felman, A. 142, 147
Fenglong (St 40) 102
fever, treatment studies 94,
   125–6
Filshie, J. 33
Fire Element (despair and
   loneliness) 84
   channel points 95–100, 203
Five Elements 81–91
   classic theory vs. hospice
      care 81–2
   concept theory and
      literature 81–2
   diagrammatic
      representation of
      sequences 82
   earth (obsessions and
      anxieties) 83–4, 91, 203
   fire (despair and
      loneliness) 84, 91, 203
   metal (denials and not
      letting go) 83, 91, 203
   water (fear and survival
      issues) 82–3, 91, 204
   wood (anger and felt
      injustices) 83, 91, 203
   overview of therapeutic
      influences 91
   use of channel points for
      93–112
Five Phases points 208
Flaws, B. 78–9
forgiveness 83
Fox, L. 115
funding
   for acupuncture treatments
      54–5, 195
   for hospice care 19–22, 29,
      36–7
   predicting care needs 55–7
Futonggu (K 20) 108
Futu (LI 18) 88, 107, 166,
   168, 175, 208

Gallbladder: Foot Shao Yang
   points 95
Garcia, M. 121–2

Gathering / Hui points 206
Gathering points 206
General Connecting Point 206
Gongsun (Sp 4) 206
Governor: Du points 112–13
grief
    emotional perspectives 63–5
    stages of 63–5
    treatments 103
gums 69
"guppy breathing" 70
gynecological conditions 74

Hale, L. 174
hands 74
harmful emotions 64–5
Harrison, I. 13–14, 43
headaches 72, 95, 97
head acupuncture 167–8, 187
head and face, diagnostic changes 66–7
head trauma 185
    see also coma
Health CMi 133, 137–8, 154–5
hearing abilities 68
Heart: Hand Shao Yin 95–6
heart attacks, studies on acupuncture use 139–40
heart disease 134–40
    hospice criteria 135
    measurement 136
    medications used 136
    patient observations 137
    stages of 135–6
heart qi deficiency 139
heart rate, diagnostic changes 75
heart yang deficiency 139
Hegu (LI 4) 84, 88–9, 94, 105–6, 121, 139, 160, 166, 168, 180, 206, 208
hepatic coma 154, 157
hepatic encephalopathy (HE) 157–9
hepatitis, safety and contamination precautions 160–1
hepatitis-B 30, 160
hepatitis-C 30

herbal medicines
    for liver disease 154–61
    see also TCM (Traditional Chinese Medicine)
herbal soba noodle soup 155–6
herpes simplex (HSV) 144
He / Uniting points 207
histoplasmosis 144
history of hospice care provisions
    China 28–30
    United States 18–23, 35–6
HIV/AIDS 29, 140–50
    hospice criteria for 140–1
    impact on immune system 141
    opportunistic infections 142–3
    other infections / diseases 143–5
    patient profiles 142–5
    TCM studies 148–50
    use of acupuncture 148–50
    use of antiretroviral drugs (ARVs) 145–7
    use of complementary therapies 147
home-based care of the dying 15–16, 22–3
    practitioners and care support aides 43, 44
home deaths
    in China 29
    with hospice support 22–3
home health aides 38–9, 43
hopelessness 111
Hopkins Technology 125–6
Hospice Acupuncture Protocol points 10, 61, 86–91
    glossary for point nomenclature 205–8
    NAHPCA treatment protocol form 201–4
Hospice Association of America 18
hospice-based deaths, data 23
Hospice by the Bay 115
hospice care
    concept described 56
    see also hospice and palliative care

Hospice of Michigan 35, 63
Hospice Minnesota for Care of the Dying 28–9
hospice nurses 43
hospice and palliative care
    accreditation 19–20
    admission criteria (general/non-specific) 188–91
    charging for 21
    concept and philosophy 13–14
    cost-effectiveness 19
    day-to-day patient management 38–9
    founding figures 16–18
    funding 19–22, 36–7, 55–7
    future trends in 35–6
    history of Chinese provisions 28–30
    history of US provisions 18–23, 35–6
    legislation for 19–22
    need for 9–11
    place of death 22–3
    referral and access 37–8
    regulation of care 19–21, 37
    role of acupuncture (overview) 32–4, 34–5, 57–61
    roles of interdisciplinary teams 43–5
    spiritual considerations 14–15
    standards of practice 19–21, 37
    therapies offered 45–7
    volunteer support 20, 36
Hospice and Palliative Care of Virginia 15
Huff, H. 150
Hui / Gathering points 206
Huizong (SJ 7) 99–100, 208
Hunmen (UB 47/42) 110
hypnotherapy 46
hypoxemia 173

infrared heat therapy 154–6
Insights of a Senior Acupuncturist (Lee) 150
insomnia 95–6, 99

insurance-based funding
    19–22, 36–7, 54–5, 195
    impact on disease
        diagnosis 119
    predicting care needs 55–7
interdisciplinary teams 42–5
itching 177, 179

jaundice 152
    skin changes 69
Jinggu (UB 64) 111–12
Jiquan (H 1) 95–6, 206
Jobst, K.A. 174–5
Johnson, S. 127
Juque (Ren / CV 14) 87–9,
    113, 139

Kanakura, Y. 124
Kaposi's sarcoma 143
Karnofsky Performance
    Scale (KPS) 190
Kasymjanova, G. 121
Kaufman, K. 33
Kemp, C. 26–9
Kidney: Foot Shao Yin
    points 107–10
kidney failure
    acute 177, 178
    chronic 177
    see also renal failure
kidneys, and pulse diagnosis
    75, 77
kidney yang deficiency 139
Kim, S. 170–2, 174
knee pain 102
Kozak, L. 60
Kübler-Ross, E. 18–19, 36,
    63–4

Lade, H. 194
Lafferty, W.E. 34
Laino, C. 149
Large Intestine: Hand Yang
    Ming points 105–7
Ledwick, M. 127
Lee, M. 150
Lee, S. 170–2, 174
legislation on hospice care
    19–22
Leng, G. 32
"letting go" 83
    acupuncture points 88–9,
        90

Lewy body dementia 131
Liangyue, D. 93
Lieque (Lu 7) 89, 103, 104–5,
    121, 123, 139, 167, 206
life expectancy, China 29
light transference in bodies
    53
Li, J. 138
limbs, diagnostic changes
    69, 74
Lingxu (K 24) 109
Lin, Y. 187
Liver: Foot Jue Yin 93–4
liver disease 150–61
    causes 152
    hospice criteria 151–2
    medication considerations
        152–3
    patient profiles 153–4
    progress of 152–3
    and Type-2 diabetes 153
    use of acupuncture 154–61
    use of specific points 160
    use of TCM 154–61
liver transplants 152
loneliness, and the Fire
    Element 84
longevity, search for 25–6
Lower He points 206
Lung: Hand Tai Yin points
    103–5
lung
    collapse 70
    see also pulmonary disease
lung cancer, treatment
    studies 121
Luo/Connecting points 206
lymphedema, treatment
    studies 124–5
Lynch, T. 9

Macicocia, G. 93
McPhail, P. 33
massage therapy 47
Master Travel Limited 30,
    31–2
meaning in life 65
Medicaid 36
medical directors 43
Medicare-certified hospices
    22, 57
    length of stay 57
    standards for 37

Medicare Hospice Benefit
    19–21, 36
    and acupuncture fees 55
medications
    Chinese herbs 150
    deaths from 26
    fear of substance addiction
        27
    see also herbal medicines;
        named substances
Melbourne Zen Hospice 34
Menter, A. 174
Meridian points see
    acupuncture points and
    meridians (overview)
Merkel cells 51
Metal Element (denials
    and not letting go) 83,
    88–9, 91
    channel points 103–7, 203
    other correspondences 91
    Yin and Yang organs 91
migraines 105
Mitchell, T. 10
Mother / Reinforcing points
    206
Mother Theresa of Calcutta
    15
motor neurone disease see
    amyotrophic lateral
    sclerosis (ALS)
mouth, diagnostic changes
    68
moxibustion
    contraindications for
        use 86
    for relieving side-effects of
        antiretroviral drugs 150
    techniques for use 86
    treatment studies 124–5,
        150
MRI scans (magnetic
    resonance imaging) 133
Mu / Collecting points 207
multiple sclerosis 164
mung beans 194
muscle tone 67
muscular atrophy 111
muscular dystrophy 163–4
music therapies 47
Myasthenia gravis 164
mycobacteria 142

National Acupuncture
    Detoxification
    Association (NADA)
    Protocol 160–1
National Hospice and
    Palliative Care
    Organization 18–19, 22,
    35–7, 40, 57
    on standards of practice 21
National Institute of Health 9
nausea 33, 60–1, 72, 98
    from chemotherapy 121
needles
    fear of 53–4
    insertion and withdrawal
        techniques 86
Neiguan (P 6) 98
neurological diseases 161–72
    forms of 161
    hospice criteria 162–3
    patient profiles 164–5
    and swallowing difficulties
        170–2
    use of acupuncture 165–72
neuroscience of acupuncture
    51–3
Nieminen, T. 25–6
Niemitzow, Richard 52
non-contact energetic
    stimulation 194
nose, diagnostic changes 67
numbness 95–6
nutritionists 44

obesity, and kidney disease
    178–9
obsessions, and the Earth
    Element 83–4
occupational therapists 45
On Death and Dying
    (Kübler-Ross) 18, 36,
    63–4

pain management 33, 60–1,
    101–6, 108, 110–12, 121,
    127, 137–8, 148–9, 165,
    167, 207–8
    fear of substance addiction
        27
    neuroscience of 51–3
pain perception, changes to
    73, 86
Pajka, S. 17–18, 65

palliative care
    concept described 55–7
    see also hospice and
        palliative care
Palliative Performance Scale
    (PPS) 38–9, 189, 190–1
Palliative Prognostic Index
    (PPI) 191
Palliative Prognostic Score
    (PaP) 191
paralysis 95–6
Parkinson's disease 164
pathoconditions 77–8
peace feelings and closure 83
performance scales for
    prognosis 38–9, 189,
    190–1
Pericardium: Hand Jue Yin
    97–9
personal care provisions
    38–9
pharmacists 44
phlegm and dampness 91,
    100, 102, 106, 158, 207,
    208
physical therapists 45
physician-assisted suicide
    20, 196–7
placebo acupuncture 124,
    174
points (general) see
    acupuncture points and
    meridians (overview)
Points of the Eight
    Extraordinary Channels
    205–6
points for fear 88
    for anger and loss feelings
        90
    for negative feelings 89
Points of Intersection 205
points for letting go 88
    for anger and loss feelings
        90
    for negative feelings 89
pressure sores 69, 184, 192–3
preventative care
    funding for 32, 55–6
    need for 55–6
Price, C. 156–7
prognosis determination
    190–1

progressive multifocal
    leukoencephalopathy
    (PML) 142–3
pruritis 179
psychiatrists 45
psychic imbalances 97–8
psychologists 45
Pucan/Pushen (UB 61) 88,
    111
Puhky, R. 81
pulmonary disease 172–5
    forms of 172
    hospice criteria 172–3
    use of acupuncture 174–5
pulse diagnosis 75–9
    contraindications for use
        84–5
    prior to death 77, 84–5
    treating chaotic pulses 85
Purushotham, A. 127

qi, growth points 207
qi-blood stagnation 139
Qimen (Liv 14) 94, 206
Qiuxu (GB 40) 88–9, 91, 95,
    166, 208
Quchi (LI 11) 89, 106, 166,
    179, 206–8
Quze (P 3) 97, 208

randomized controlled trials
    (RCTs)
    on Asian Medicine 33, 150
    ethical considerations
        123–4
regulation of care 19–21, 37
Reisberg, B. 128–9
renal failure 175–80
    hospice criteria 175–8
    patient profiles 178–9
    use of acupuncture studies
        179–80
renal function, use of
    acupuncture studies 180
research and cost
    effectiveness
    Asian Medicine practices
        31–2
    neuroscience of
        acupuncture 51–3
    use of acupuncture in
        hospice care 34–5,
        58–61, 195

use with cancer patients
121–7
use of RCTs in palliative
care patients 123–4
and WHO resources 195
respite care 39
restlessness 66
Rhubarb 159
right heart failure (RHF) 173
Ritchie, H. 40–1
Roger, M. 40–1
Romeo, M.J. 60
Rubens, C. 33

sacrum, skin discolorations
69
St. Christopher's Hospice
(London) 16–17
St. John, T. 30, 31
salivation difficulties 96, 98
Salkeld, E.J. 33
San Jiao: Hand Shao Yang
99–100, 205
Sanyinjiao (Sp 6) 89, 101,
121, 124–5, 155, 157,
179, 205
Saunders, Cicely Mary
16–17, 199
scalp acupuncture 167–8,
187
Schwartz, G. 148
Schwartz, M. 44
sciatica 111
sclera 67
Sea of Marrow point 207
Sea points 207
*The Secret of Chinese Pulse
Diagnosis* (Flaws) 78–9
Sedation / Reducing point
207
self-absorption feelings 83–4
sensory organs, and the Five
Elements 91
septicemia 193–4
Shanghai College of
Traditional Medicine 93
Shencang (K 25) 109–10
Shenfeng (K 23) 109
Shengtang (UB 44/39) 110
Shenmen (H 7) 87, 96, 121,
123, 138–9, 207–8
Shiflett, S. 148
Shui / Water points 208

Shu / Transporting points
207
Silberstein, Morry 51–2
The Simple Questions
(Chinese medical book)
65–6
Sishencong points 113
skin, diagnostic changes
69, 74
sleep, changes in 73
Small Intestine: Hand Tai
Yang 96–7
smells, body odours 71
social workers 43
Soh, K. 52
Sommers, E. 148–9
Son points 207
Sontang Caring Hospital
(Beijing) 28–9
soups 155–6
speech and language
therapists 45
the spirit of a person 65–6
accessing 83
spirit points 85, 87, 207–8
for anger feelings 90
for negative feelings and
fears 89
spiritual chaos 94, 105
spiritual considerations
14–15
and cultural burial
practices 27–8
Spleen: Foot Tai Yin 100–1
standards of practice
history of 19–21
for hospices 37
for pediatric palliative
care 21
Standish, L.J. 60
Stanrock, J. 65
sthenia syndromes 126
Stomach: Foot Yang Ming
101–3
stools, changes to 71, 73
stroke 180–7
causes 180
forms of 182–3
hospice criteria 181–2
progress of 183–4
signs and symptoms 183–4
Strong, K. 29
Sudhakaran, P. 166, 169
Su Wen book 81

Suzuki, M. 174–5
swallowing difficulties 69,
72–3, 170–2, 184
sweating 72

Taibai (Sp 3) 100, 168, 171,
207–8
Taichong (Liv 3) 84, 88–9,
93–4, 121, 139, 155, 160,
207–8
Taixi (K 3) 88, 107–8, 139,
155, 157, 168, 175,
179–80, 207–8
Taiyuan (Lu 9) 88, 105, 139,
171, 175, 206–8
Tangcao tablets 150
Taoism 26
taste, and the Five Elements
91
TCM (Traditional Chinese
Medicine) 31–2
and cancer symptom
classifications 123
use in heart disease 137–40
use in liver disease 154–61
see also Asian Medicine
TDP heat lamps 155–6
teeth and gums, diagnostic
changes 68
terminal illness (general/
non-specific) 57, 188–94
the last treatment 194
prognosis determination
190–1
Therrien, A. 126–7
thirst, loss of 73
throat, diagnostic changes 69
Tianding (LI 17) 88, 106
Tianfu (Lu 3) 104, 208
Tianjing (SJ 10) 100, 207–8
Tianzong (SI 11) 96–7, 205
Tibetan Medicine, on
harmful emotions 65
tinnitus 73
tongue, diagnostic changes
68
toxoplasmosis 143
Traditional Chinese
Medicine (TCM), scope
of 31–2
Transporting / Shu points
207
tuberculosis 29, 145
Tu / Earth points 208

Type-2 diabetes 137
    and kidney failure 176,
        178–9
    and liver disease 153

ulcers 184, 192–3
UNAIDS 142
United States
    healthcare system 31, 32
    healthcare expenditure 40
    history of hospice care
        provision 18–23, 35–6
    home-based deaths 39–40
    mortality causes 40–1
    number of hospices 40
    population data 39
    population health profiles
        39–42
United States Census Bureau
    10, 39
Unschuld, P. 65–6, 75
uremic pruritus 179
Urinary Bladder: Foot Tai
    Yang points 110–12
urine, changes to 71, 73

veterans health care 20, 55
Viera, F.M. 170
viral load 141
Vlasto, T. 52–3
voice, changes to 70

volunteer support 20, 36, 44
vomiting 35, 60, 97, 109, 110,
    122, 170, 197

Wald, Florence 17–18
Wang, J. 150
Water Element (fear and
    survival issues) 82–3,
    88, 91
    channel points 107–12, 204
weight loss 191–2
Wei, Li 28
Window to the Sky points
    208
Wong, M. 26–7
Wood Element (anger and
    felt injustices) 83, 88, 91
    channel points 93–5, 203
World Health Organization
    9, 49, 58–60, 118, 195
    on role of acupuncture
        therapies 34, 195
Wu Xing / Element points
    208

xenobiotic detoxes 156–7
xerostomia, treatment
    studies 123–4
Xi / Cleft point 97, 99, 208
Xie, H. 139
Ximen (P 4) 97–8, 138, 208
Xu, L. 138

Yangchi (SJ 4) 99, 208
Yang, J. 192–3
Yanglingquan (GB 34) 160,
    167–8, 186, 186–7
Yang organs, and the Five
    Elements 91
yang qi collapse 140
Yao, C. 157–9
The Yellow Emperor's Classic
    of Internal Medicine
    75–6, 81
yin deficiency 139–40
Yin organs, and the Five
    Elements 91
Youmen (K 21) 108–9, 205
Yuan Source point 208
Yu, J. 180

Zhang, C. 137
Zhangmen (Liv 13) 89–90,
    94, 205–7
Zhishi (UB 52/47) 111, 208
Zhongfu (Lu 1) 103–4, 175,
    205–7
Zou, W. 150
Zusanli (St 36) 89, 101–2,
    121, 123–5, 138–40, 149,
    160, 166–8, 170, 175,
    179–80, 206–8

Thank you for your purchase of *Hospice and Palliative Care Acupuncture*. Your purchase of this material supports the efforts of the National Association of Hospice and Palliative Care Acupuncturists (NAHPCA) to help educate hospice organizations and train acupuncture professionals in end-of-life care. We believe when we all give a little we all gain a lot. To learn more about the NAHPCA, visit our website: www.nahpca.com.

You will also find information on our many levels of membership, and how to become a Certified Provider of Hospice and Palliative Care Acupuncture (CPHPCA).

CPI Antony Rowe
Eastbourne, UK
September 29, 2023